Guidelines for
Clinical Nursing
Practices

Related to a Nursing Model

Elizabeth M. Jamieson RGN ONC RCT RNT
Janice M. McCall BA RGN RCT
Rona Blythe SRN SCM RCT RNT

Clinical Lecturers, Department of Health and Nursing Studies, Glasgow Polytechnic

Winifred W. Logan MA DNS (Educ) RGN RNT

Consultant

SECOND EDITION

Churchill Livingstone 🏛

EDINBURGH LONDON MADRID MELBOURNE NEW YORK AND TOKYO 1992

CHURCHILL LIVINGSTONE
Medical Division of Longman Group UK Limited

Distributed in the United States of America by Churchill
Livingstone Inc., 650 Avenue of the Americas, New York,
N. Y. 10011, and by associated companies, branches and
representatives throughout the world.

First edition 1988
Second edition 1992
  Reprinted 1993

ISBN 0-443-04440-6

British Library Cataloguing in Publication Data
A catalogue record for this book is available from the British
Library.

Library of Congress Cataloging in Publication Data
Jamieson, Elizabeth M. (Elizabeth Marion)
  Guidelines for clinical nursing practices: related to a
  nursing model/Elizabeth M. Jamieson, Janice M. McCall,
  Rona Blythe; Winifred W. Logan, consultant. – – 2nd ed.
    p.   cm.
  Includes bibliographical references and index.
  ISBN (invalid) 0–433–04440–6
  1. Nursing — Handbooks, manuals, etc. I. McCall, Janice M.
  II. Blythe, Rona. III. Logan, Winifred W. IV. Title. V. Title:
  Clinical nursing practices.
  [DNLM: 1. Nursing Care — handbooks. WY 39 J32g]
RT51.J38 1992
610.73 — dc20
DNLM/DLC
for Library of Congress   90-20501
                                           CIP

The
publisher's
policy is to use
**paper manufactured
from sustainable forests**

Produced by Longman Singapore Publishers (Pte) Ltd
Printed in Singapore

Preface

This book is concerned with selected nursing practices or interventions. The selection of practices was made with the aim of including all those which the non-specialist nurse should be able to perform safely.

By 'nursing practice' we mean the intervention itself, devised in response to assessing a patient's problems and making a nursing plan. It encompasses the thinking processes which are required before, during and after each nursing intervention. In addition, there is information on follow-up and evaluation of outcome.

We feel that a book of this kind is required now more than ever, both for those just starting their nursing studies and for the many individuals returning to nursing after a career break. It is a book which attempts to establish clearly in the student's mind, from the outset of his or her career (or, indeed, when that career is resumed), the *crucial link* between theory and practice, and the equally important concept that these apparently physical nursing practices require psychosocial skills just as much as manual dexterity. These two aims have been kept firmly in mind throughout the book.

The main title of the book, *Guidelines for Clinical Nursing Practices*, was chosen with care and is significant. They are guidelines as to what the nurse should do when he or she is carrying out a nurse-initiated intervention, such as a bed bath; or helping the medical practitioner to carry out, for example, a lumbar puncture. The guidelines are succinct and stress principles, since the detail of practice inevitably varies from one place to another. At the same time, they give much more information than can usually be found in larger textbooks of nursing.

In another sense, too, they are guidelines, in that students are expected and encouraged to consult other texts for background knowledge. At the end of each nursing practice there is a suggested reading list, and relevant research reports are included. Most of the references, in turn, provide further suggestions for reading about the particular topic. This should encourage students to seek knowledge from a number of sources, to learn about research findings, to understand why they carry out a nursing practice and to see the actual intervention as one very important part (but still only a part) of a total plan of care.

The subtitle, *Related to a Nursing Model*, is equally significant. The nursing practices have been viewed within the framework of a model for nursing which includes the process of nursing. Although the book can be used in combination with any model, one has been selected throughout to provide the student with examples of its application — the Roper, Logan and Tierney model for nursing as described in *The Elements of Nursing* (1990). The importance we attach to this link with a nursing model cannot be over-emphasised: the nursing practices are described according to how they influence various Activities of Living (ALs); they are grouped in the Contents according to the main AL they affect; and guidelines for evaluation of outcome are grouped under other relevant ALs. Essentially, the reference is to the patient's ALs, but when relevant the nurse's responsibilities are also categorised according to ALs —for example, under Maintaining a Safe Environment, there is reference to the nurse's responsibility to all patients, to him or herself and to other staff in observing the general principles related to the prevention of cross-infection.

We appreciate that a book of this type is not normally read from beginning to end in one sitting. Rather, we expect that it will be referred to on many different occasions, when the student wants to understand the practice in the context of a total plan of care which must be performed safely. It will also depend on what the individual nurse is doing or studying at the time, so that the order in which the practices will be read will inevitably vary. This means that, in many cases, there is repetition: for example, 'ensuring privacy' is mentioned under many different practices, but we feel such repetition is not only justified but essential. We have also relied on cross-references to other practices, to ensure that essential points are not passed over or assumed.

However, there are some general points about the philosophy underlying this book, how it is structured and why, which we felt had to be stated clearly, in a certain amount of detail, and at the beginning. This has been done in Part 1, the Introduction, and *we urge all users of this book to read the Introduction with care and reflection, before going on to the practices themselves*. Not to do so would be to lose the full benefit of this text.

We anticipate that this book will be used in a variety of settings — in the practice area, in the school or college, or for private study. We have therefore included illustrations which will enhance the book's value wherever it is used, but in particular away from the ward itself. In this way it should be an invaluable tool for students engaged in self-learning or experiential-based programmes.

We also expect that the book will be consulted by students at various stages of their basic nurse education programme — indeed, probably throughout their course and after qualification as well. We have therefore tried to ensure that the information is written at a level suitable for even the more junior student, but with the understanding that all students must be willing and able to consult supplementary texts on relevant sciences such as physiology, anatomy, psychology and sociology, and in the humanities.

Of course, the material may be used differently depending on the level of the user's nursing experience. Benner (1984, p. 1), applying to nursing the Dreyfus model of skill acquisition, outlines five levels of proficiency — novice, advanced beginner, competent, proficient and expert — indicating the different modes of using theoretical knowledge as the novice becomes more experienced. Whereas the novice, as a *detached observer*, takes note of what appear to be 'separate' entities in a nursing skill, there is progression towards becoming an *informed performer* who sees the situation as a 'whole'.

Finally, we should say a bit about ourselves: the authors are three clinical lecturers who are involved, daily, with students in a nursing degree programme. We have a wealth of experience in applying theory in a practice setting in the day-to-day bustle of a group of hospitals. Indeed, rather than teaching students, we try to 'help them to learn' about nursing by linking theoretical skills and manual dexterity. As we said before, we feel this book is urgently needed, but the content can only be useful if the student engages in the cognitive skills which are required before, during and after each nursing intervention.

We are convinced that high standards of observable nursing practice and thinking are intimately bound together: we hope that this book will assist nurses to provide patients/clients with a standard of nursing practice which is professionally satisfying, and which the public deserve.

Glasgow, 1992   EJ, JMcC and RB

REFERENCE

Benner P 1984 From novice to expert: excellence and power in clinical nursing practice. Addison–Wesley Publishing Company, Menlo Park, California

Alphabetical List of Nursing Practices

Contents

Part 1

Introduction

Introduction

Over a hundred years ago, Florence Nightingale argued that good nursing must contain a strong 'thinking' as well as a 'doing' component. 'Observation tells us the facts, reflection tells us the meaning of the fact... observation tells us how the patient is, reflection tells us what is to be done'.

Unfortunately, many people still think of nursing as a series of tasks. They do not realise that, as well as possessing manual skills, nurses need knowledge and the ability to think and reflect about a task if it is to be done effectively.

This book has been written to further the aim, alluded to by Nightingale, of integrating theory and practice in nursing. As was stated in the Preface, the focus of the book is nursing practices, by which is meant not simply the tasks themselves but also the thinking which surrounds them.

The purpose of this Introduction, which we hope all users of the book will read before going on to Part 2 on the practices, is:

- to provide the student with a brief introduction to the theoretical background of the book and refer them to the more substantial texts on the subject for further study

- to explain the relationship between nursing models, in particular the Roper, Logan and Tierney model for nursing, and the content of this book

- to summarise briefly the main headings used for each practice in Part 2 and what each heading covers

The theoretical background in nursing

This book is necessary because, unfortunately, not only the public think of nursing as a series of tasks. Despite the Nightingale emphasis on the need for a combination of cognitive skills and manual dexterity, the theme of 'functional orientation' has persisted in the nursing profession itself. Loomis (1974) defines 'functional orientation' as being busy doing procedures rather than thinking, reflecting and problem-solving, and maintains that this orientation originates from the early inclusion of nurse training programmes in hospital settings which socialised nurses into being intellectually subordinate. So, she goes on, as a group they developed an attitude of task orientation, and nursing has remained at a practical level only, rather than developing a theoretical level on which to base the practice. Despite this indictment, there have been many nurses who did not consider that 'doing' and 'thinking' were mutually exclusive; who have struggled to emphasise the need for identifying the theoretical base for practice, and have eschewed blind obedience to ritual, routine and unquestioning tradition.

The development of nursing models

During the last 3 decades, a number of nurse writers and practitioners have published their attempts to identify the theoretical base of nursing. Some have undertaken research to corroborate their hypotheses. Particularly of late there has been healthy debate about which comes first – do theories grow out of what nursing is and how nurses deliver care, or is a theoretical framework developed first, providing guidelines for the practice?

In pursuit of theory development, certain writers have attempted to clarify their thinking by using a model for nursing (the term 'conceptual framework' is sometimes used) as an intermediate step to theory development.

Fawcett (1984), discussing models from a variety of disciplines, maintains that each evolved from the empirical observations and intuitive insights of scholars, and/or deductions that creatively combine ideas from several fields of enquiry. However, she goes on, each model includes only those concepts which the model-builders considered a relevant representation of the real world, and an aid to understanding.

Using models has certainly come to be part of the search for the knowledge base of nursing. Of course, models are useful in any discipline as a visual representation of its theoretical framework. They indicate the main concepts, and just as importantly, show the relationship between the concepts – even when these relationships have not yet been rigorously tested by research. Each model is one person's individual interpretation of the discipline, offered as an aid to further thinking, and is a growing point.

To concentrate on thinking to the exclusion of nursing practice, of course, is folly. Nursing is a practice discipline. However, as McFarlane noted (1986, p. 1) 'practice shorn of any theoretical basis and which does not allow its theoretical foundation to grow is not a practice discipline. It is a ritualised performance . . .'.

Types of nursing models

It is not possible or desirable here to argue the finer points of nursing theory or to discuss in detail the best-known models for nursing. There are numerous texts on the subject and some of these are listed at the end of the Introduction. Suffice it to say that nursing models can be grouped into categories which indicate their major thrust. McFarlane (1986, p. 4) suggests four main types:

- interaction models (Travelbee 1971, Riehl 1980, Orlando 1961, King 1981)

- developmental models related to lifespan (Peplau 1952, Thibodeau 1983)

- self-care, activities of living, and human needs models (Henderson 1966, Rogers 1970, Orem 1985, Roper, Logan & Tierney 1990)

- system models (Roy 1980)

It should also be noted that all of the named model-builders use a person-centred model and all, in some form or other, include the following in their interpretation:

- the concept of interaction

- the concept of development

- the concept of man as part of an open system with a dynamic interplay

- between the individual and his environment

- some form of recognition of the individual's lifestyle

And yet, despite these similarities, it must also be acknowledged that when a particular model is chosen to guide practice, it does influence the form of the assessment which is used and the way in which the documentation of the nursing plan is presented.

The relationship of this book to nursing models

This book has been written with examples related to one particular model for nursing – the Roper, Logan and Tierney model – although the content can be used along with any other model. The Roper, Logan and Tierney model was selected because for eight years the authors of this book, all clinical lecturers, have been using it successfully in the practice setting with students on a degree programme for nursing. These same students also learn to apply other models for nursing in the practice setting, but because the Roper, Logan and Tierney model is so readily understandable by learners, it was selected for use in this book.

Roper, Logan and Tierney present their model in full in their book *The Elements of Nursing* (1990), which students are urged to study carefully. The Roper, Logan and Tierney model, it should be recalled, has five main concepts:

- activities of living (ALs)

- lifespan

- dependence–independence continuum

- factors related to ALs:
  — physical
  — psychological
  — sociocultural (including spiritual/religious and ethical)
  — environmental
  — politicoeconomic (including legal)

- individuality and individualising nursing
  — assessing
  — planning
  — implementing
  — evaluating

These five concepts and the relationships between them have to be considered when making a nursing plan, and therefore when carrying out a nursing practice which is part of that plan. The following three examples should illustrate this point.

Example 1

The important nursing action of explaining to the patient (and family when appropriate) what will occur during an intervention, and seeking consent and cooperation, relates to the AL of Communicating. At face value, this activity may seem to involve merely the physical action of listening and talking. But of course there are important psychological and sociocultural considerations, for example choosing language suited to the patient's age (stage of the lifespan), degree of dependence/independence, and sociocultural background. The related non-verbal communication is also important, and includes more than the simple physical manifestation of 'talking'. Sometimes communicating may mean helping the patient adjust to changes in his usual lifestyle, which may involve psychological, sociocultural, environmental and politicoeconomic factors.

Example 2

Isolation nursing also shows clearly that nursing practices are much more than merely physical tasks. Washing hands and safely disposing of used equipment are patently physical activities which relate to the AL of Maintaining a Safe Environment. However, psychological and social factors feature importantly in isolation nursing: for example, ensuring that the patient does not feel alone when 'reverse barrier nursing' is required; or, in 'barrier nursing', avoiding feelings of being ostracised or stigmatised on the patient's part because his eating and sanitary utensils are kept separate from those of other patients, and his clothing and body discharges are handled by individuals with gloved hands. Nursing someone with HIV gives rise also to important ethical considerations, an aspect which has been well publicised recently in the professional literature and the mass media.

Example 3

In almost every nursing practice, the patient's privacy is mentioned – the need to protect the patient's privacy; to preserve dignity; to prevent embarrassment; to be sensitive to the patient's anxiety because of even a temporary change in body image such as the presence of a catheter or a stoma bag. Using bed screens and covering the patient as much as possible are physical activities, but there are also psychological and sociocultural considerations related for example to the AL of Expressing Sexuality, i.e. femininity, masculinity.

These three examples highlight the importance of the decision to relate the nursing practices to a nursing model. It should ensure the following:

- that the patient's individuality is always uppermost in the nurse's mind

- that important aspects of nursing which relate to (but are not part of) the physical activity itself are not omitted

- that the theoretical basis of all nursing practices is not forgotten – the base both in nursing theory and in other disciplines such as the physical and social sciences and the humanities

Finally, there are two further ways in which the link between the nursing practices and the Roper, Logan and Tierney model has been made apparent:

- The nursing practices are discussed within the framework of the 12 ALs as used in the Roper, Logan and Tierney model for nursing.

- The nursing practices are grouped, in the Contents, under the 12 ALs (they can also be found alphabetically in the list at the beginning of the book).

This use of the ALs is quite purposeful: it is hoped that it will reinforce in the student's mind the relationship of the nursing practices to the broader theoretical base.

The nursing practices: the main headings

Knowing that this book would be 'dipped into' rather than read from cover to cover, as we stated in the Preface, we felt it was important to present the information for each practice in a consistent format. This should allow the student to use the book easily and quickly, once he or she has become familiar with the way in which the material is presented and, in particular, what can be found under the main headings used for each practice. These are:

- Objectives
- Related information
- Some indications for ...
- Outline of the procedure
- Equipment
- Guidelines for this nursing practice
- Relevance to the activities of living
- Suggested reading

A brief summary is given below of the material covered under each of these headings.

Introduction

Objectives

The material under this heading indicates what the student should know after reading and studying this practice, in combination with his or her existing personal knowledge and knowledge from other sources – the physical and social sciences, the humanities, professional nursing literature.

It is, of course, necessary for nursing staff (teaching and clinical) to demonstrate to the student the manual aspects of the practice.

Related information

Included here are suggested areas of physiology and anatomy which should be reviewed to promote safe manual practice. Knowledge of physical aspects is emphasised here because the practices described in the book are physical tasks and must be performed safely. (The relationship of psychosocial theory to the physical practice, and the importance of combining the two, are dealt with more fully under the subsequent heading 'Relevance to the activities of living'.)

In addition, cross-references to related nursing practices are given here, and the student's attention is also drawn to the need to consult health authority policy, if it is likely to have a particular bearing on this practice.

Some indications for ...

Under this heading a definition of the nursing practice is given, where relevant, and common disease conditions, or other instances for which the practice might be undertaken, are mentioned. It was deliberately decided *not* to give a definition at the beginning of each practice, but rather to place it in its context – that is, alongside examples of circumstances which may give rise to the practice. Definitions given in isolation may lead to the mistaken view that the nursing practices are tasks with a beginning and an end, rather than part of a nursing plan which requires thought and reflection.

Outline of the procedure

This heading appears for those few procedures normally performed by a medical practitioner, where the nurse is present to nurse the patient and/or assist the medical staff (a part of nursing which is 'doctor-initiated'). It gives a brief description of the sequence of events, so that the nursing student can follow the steps intelligently; usually includes information about the position of the patient during the procedure; describes some of the commonly used tests; and emphasises the role of the nurse. 'Outline of the procedure' may also appear if a particular theory needs to be highlighted.

Equipment

The material under this heading is virtually a list of the equipment commonly used for the particular nursing practice. As far as possible, general terms such as 'local anaesthetic' or 'water-based lotion for cleansing the skin' are used, and specific brand names are merely cited as examples. Where appropriate, some equipment is described, for example the different types of catheter used in urinary catheterisation; the types of packaging used for IV infusions and how they are connected to the infusion system; the various parts of the lumbar puncture needle.

In many instances, diagrams or drawings of actual pieces of equipment are given to supplement the text.

Guidelines for this nursing practice

The general principles for the practice are outlined here, and the following points should be noted.

Near the beginning of the guidelines, the student is alerted to 'observe the patient throughout the nursing practice': some suggested observations are given under the subsequent heading 'Relevance to the activities of living'.

At the end of the guidelines, there is a statement 'document the nursing practice appropriately, observe after-effects and report abnormal findings immediately'. The meaning attached to these three phrases is discussed below:

— The wording '*document each nursing practice appropriately*' was chosen carefully: discussion of methods of documentation would merit a separate book, and therefore has not been attempted here. In each ward, clinic or community setting, a method of documentation will have been decided upon; indeed, in some authorities nursing data are recorded on computers.
— '*Observe after-effects*' is really a follow-on to the earlier guideline 'observe the patient throughout the nursing practice': it is part of the process of evaluating outcome – an integral phase of the process of nursing (individualising nursing).
— '*Report abnormal findings immediately*' alerts the student to the need, not just to document the practice, but to report abnormal findings immediately to the nurse in charge: abnormal findings often require immediate action, for example, altering the site of an IV infusion needle when there is evidence of fluid infiltrating the tissues around the site; discontinuing a drug because of the appearance of a rash; investigating the cause of pain in the calf of the leg following surgery, which can be indicative of deep venous thrombosis.

Relevance to the activities of living

Observing is a crucial part of nursing, and Nightingale comments on its importance in the quotation given at the beginning of this Introduction. However, rather than giving a list of observations to be made before, during and after each nursing practice, the authors thought it would be much more helpful to present observations as and when they related – and only when they *directly* related – to the ALs suggested in the Roper, Logan and Tierney model for nursing. Usually the reference is to the patient's ALs, but when relevant, the nurse's responsibilities are also given by AL. For example, under Maintaining a Safe Environment, there is reference to the nurse's responsibility to all patients, to him or herself and to other members of staff in observing the general principles for preventing cross-infection.

Moreover, whereas under the second heading 'Related information', material on the physical aspects of each practice is cited (because the content of the book is essentially concerned with observable physical procedures which must be carried out safely) this AL section *combines* physical science knowledge with the psychosocial and humanities knowledge which must be used before, during and after each nursing practice. It is this integrated thinking process which differentiates the performance of a routine; physical task – even when performed dexterously – from a nursing practice. It demands assessment, planning and evaluation related to the specific practice within the context of the patient's total plan of care. Each nursing practice is an important part (but still only a part) of a total nursing plan.

Introduction

Suggested reading This list includes books, articles and research reports relevant to each nursing practice, where available and most references provide suggestions for further reading around the topic. This guided search and self-search is intended to encourage students to look at a variety of sources, to learn about research findings and to understand the reason behind specific practices in the context of a total care plan.

In addition, the authors assume that students are using supplementary texts in related fields such as the sciences and humanities. Also to gain full benefit from this book, the beginning student should be conversant with *The Elements of Nursing* (Roper, Logan & Tierney 1990).

In conclusion, we hope that this Introduction will provide a thought-provoking foundation for the nursing practices which follow. As stated in the Preface, the practices are as succinct as possible for ease of reference and we are confident that readers who assimilate the principles outlined in the Introduction will be able to utilise the practices with individuality — while respecting the patient's special needs — and with the depth of thought which all nursing actions deserve and, indeed, should demand.

It is important to emphasise too that, apart from maintaining a legal record, well-charted practices and observations are essential in developing nursing theory. In fact, Benner (1984, p. 11) goes further and maintains that the practices and expertise of good nurse clinicians contain a wealth of untapped knowledge, which will not expand unless nurses systematically record for themselves what they learn from their own practice experience.

References and suggested reading

Benner P 1984 From novice to expert: excellence and power in clinical nursing practice. Addison Wesley, Menlo Park, California

Fawcett J 1984 Analysis and evaluation of conceptual models of nursing. F A Davis, Philadelphia, p 4

Fraser M 1990 Using conceptual nursing in practice: a research-based approach. Harper and Row, London

Henderson V 1966 The nature of nursing. Macmillan, New York

King I 1981 A theory for nursing: systems concept process. John Wiley, New York

Loomis M 1974 Collegiate nursing education: an ambivalent professionalism. In: Meleis A (ed) 1985 Theoretical nursing: development and progress. Lippincott, Philadelphia, p 38

McFarlane J 1986 The value of models for care. In: Kershaw B, Salvage J (eds) Models for nursing. John Wiley, New York, pp 1–6

Meleis A 1985 Theoretical nursing: development and progress. Lippincott, Philadelphia

Orem D 1985 Nursing: concepts of practice. McGraw-Hill, New York

Orlando I 1961 The dynamic nurse–patient relationship: function, process and principles. Pitman, New York

Pearson A, Vaughan B 1986 Nursing models for practice. Heinemann, London

Peplau H 1952 Interpersonal relations in nursing. Pitman, New York

Riehl J 1980 in Riehl J, Roy C (eds) Conceptual models for nursing practice. Appleton-Century-Crofts, Norwalk

Rogers M 1970 An introduction to the theoretical basis of nursing. F A Davis, Philadelphia

Roper N, Logan W, Tierney A 1990 The elements of nursing, 3rd edn. Churchill Livingstone, Edinburgh

Roy C 1980 In: Riehl J, Roy C (eds) Conceptual models for nursing practice. Appleton-Century-Crofts, Norwalk

Thibodeau J 1983 Nursing models: analysis and evaluation. Wadsworth Health Sciences Division, Monterey, California

Travelbee J 1971 Interpersonal aspects of nursing. F A Davis, Philadelphia

Wright S 1986 Building and using a model for nursing. Edward Arnold, London

Part 2

The Nursing Practices

Section 1

Maintaining a
Safe Environment

Administration of Medicines

Objectives

By the end of this section you should know how to:

- prepare the patient for this nursing practice
- collect the equipment
- carry out administration of medicines

Related information

Review of the Misuse of Drugs Act 1971 with special reference to the storage and administration of drugs.

Review of health authority policy regarding the patient's medicine prescription and recording documents, and disposal of equipment used.

Revision of the pharmacology of the medication to be administered.

Revision of the metric system of volume and weight used in a dose calculation of a medication.

Review of United Kingdom Central Council for Nursing, Midwifery and Health Visiting advisory paper on administration of medicines 1986 and circular on administration of medicines 1988.

Some indications for administration of medicines

A medication can be administered by a variety of routes and for many different reasons:

- to alleviate pain or discomfort caused by disease, injury or surgery
- to prevent disease
- to alleviate a manifestation of disease
- to cure disease

Equipment

Patient's medicine prescription and recording documents

Medication to be administered

Equipment for use during medicine administration, e.g.:
— oral administration: medicine glass or spoon, jug of water, patient's glass
— injection: appropriately-sized sterile needle and syringe, alcohol saturated swab for skin cleansing

Trolley or tray for equipment

Receptacle for soiled disposables

Guidelines for this nursing practice

All forms of medicine administration

- explain the nursing practice to the patient and gain his consent and cooperation*
- wash the hands
- collect and prepare the equipment
- ensure the patient's privacy
- observe the patient throughout this activity
- identify the medicine to be administered on the patient's prescription document. The prescription should be complete, correct and legible
- check that the medicine has not already been administered
- select the appropriate medicine against the prescription document
- check the medicine name, dosage and expiry date

- remove the prescribed dosage from the container
- check the prescription and dosage against the medicine container
- identify the patient to whom the medicine is to be administered by checking his identification bracelet unit number and when appropriate by verbal verification by the patient against the details on his prescription document
- administer the medicine by the route prescribed
- ensure that the patient is left feeling as comfortable as possible
- dispose of the equipment safely
- document the nursing practice appropriately, monitor after-effects and report abnormal findings immediately

Controlled drugs

The administration of a controlled drug within a hospital environment must involve two nurses, one of whom is a registered nurse practitioner. A controlled drug register is kept on each ward or department giving details of the stock and administration of controlled drugs.

- as for all forms of medicine administration to the Guideline which ends '... not already been administered'
- remove the appropriate medicine from the controlled drug store, check the stock number with the number detailed in the register with the other nurse
- check the date of the prescription
- check the method of administration
- check the time of administration

- remove the appropriate dose from the stock of controlled drugs, checking the name and dosage with the second nurse. Check the stock number of the remaining controlled drugs
- enter into the controlled drug register the appropriate details
- continue as for all forms of medicine administration

*To maintain brevity in the practices, we have in general used 'he' for the patient and 'she' for the nurse.

Administration of Medicines

Guidelines for this
nursing practice
continued

Oral preparations

- as for all forms of medicine administration to the Guideline which begins 'remove the prescribed dosage...'

- remove required number of *tablets, pills* or *cachets* from medicine container without contaminating the preparation. Place into the medicine glass or medicine spoon

  or

- shake the *liquid* medicine preparation well. Pour into the appropriate container at eye level and on a solid flat surface

- check the medicine prescription and dosage against the container

- identify the patient

- administer the medicine, offer the patient a drink of water to aid administration of the oral preparation if allowed

- continue as for all forms of medicine administration

Injection preparations

- as for all forms of medicine administration to the Guideline which ends '... checking the drug name, dosage and expiry date'

- assemble the appropriate-sized needle and syringe, maintaining asepsis

- prepare the fluid for injection as recommended by the manufacturer

- withdraw the appropriate amount of solution in relation to the medicine dose prescribed

- identify the patient to whom the medicine is to be administered

- ensure the patient's privacy

- expose the chosen site for intramuscular injection (Fig. 1.1) or subcutaneous injection (Fig. 1.2)

Figure 1.1
Administration of medicines: sites used for intramuscular injection
A Upper outer quadrant of the buttock
B Anterior lateral aspect of the thigh
C Deltoid region of the arm

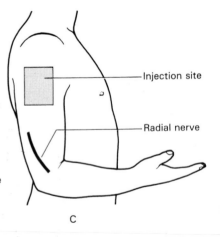

Injection site

Radial nerve

Injection site

Sciatic nerve

A

C

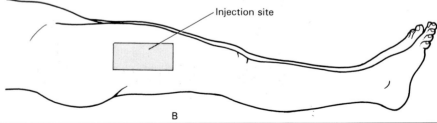

Injection site

B

- cleanse the skin using the alcohol-saturated swab

- for an intramuscular injection, using the non-dominant hand stretch the skin over the site. With the dominant hand introduce 2/3 of the needle at a 90° angle to the skin

- for a subcutaneous injection using the non-dominant hand gently grip the skin over the site. With the dominant hand introduce 2/3 of the needle at a 45° angle to the skin

- withdraw the piston of the syringe; if blood is drawn up into the syringe withdraw the needle and syringe from the patient's tissue. Replace the needle and start again

- if no blood is withdrawn into the syringe inject the solution slowly

- withdraw the needle smoothly and quickly. Apply pressure to the site of injection if bleeding occurs

- continue as for all forms of medicine administration

Topical applications

For instillation of eyedrops and ointment (see pp. 55–57)
For instillation of eardrops (see p. 50)

Rectal and vaginal preparations

For instillation of a rectal suppository and an enema (see pp. 220–222)
For instillation of a vaginal pessary (see p. 308)

Preparations by inhalation

For inhalation of a medicine (see p. 98)
For a medicine administered by a nebuliser (see p. 94)

Figure 1.2
Administration of medicines: sites used for subcutaneous injection
A Anterior aspect
B Posterior aspect

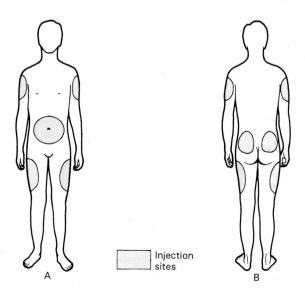

Injection sites

A

B

Administration of Medicines

Maintaining a safe environment

The nurse in charge of a ward or department at any time of the day or night is responsible for maintaining the safe and correct storage of all medications held within that ward or department. The storage requirements are enforced by law through the Misuse of Drugs Act 1971. All records pertaining to medicine administration must be maintained adhering to health authority legal requirements.

A learner nurse should be supervised by a qualified member of staff while administering medicines. In hospital a nurse can only administer a medicine on the written instruction of a medical practitioner unless she works in a specialised unit such as an intensive care unit. The medicine prescription should be written in indelible ink, giving the date, patient's full name and age, the medication name (preferably generic title), dosage to be given, time of administration, and must be signed by a medical practitioner. The whole prescription should be legible.

The nurse is responsible for the correct administration and documentation of a prescribed medication. Recording of the administration may only be performed once the nurse is satisfied that the patient has received the prescribed medication. Should any error occur during administration this must be reported so that the appropriate action can be implemented.

The manufacturer's recommendations for the storage environment and expiry date should be adhered to otherwise the medicine composition may be altered.

The nurse should familiarise herself with the use, action, common side-effects and therapeutic dose of the medication she administers. This will help her to educate the patient about the medication and identify any adverse reaction the patient may develop.

Oral medicine administration does not require aseptic technique but all equipment should be clean or disposable and all precautions taken to prevent cross-infection. The nurse should wash her hands before commencing and on completion of oral medicine administration.

When a patient has difficulty in swallowing an oral preparation the nurse may request the medicine to be supplied in another form. Tablets if scored can be halved to achieve the prescribed dose. Pills, capsules and cachets should be supplied in the dosage stated on the prescription sheet.

Oral liquids should be shaken well prior to pouring the prescribed amount, to thoroughly disperse the medicine in the liquid base. Any spillage down the outside of the bottle should be wiped off to prevent disfiguration of the label.

As an injection is an invasive procedure all principles of asepsis should be maintained. The equipment should then be disposed of safely and immediately following the injection to reduce the potential hazards. Certain medications can be hazardous to staff during preparation and administration, therefore disposable gloves may be required.

An intramuscular injection should only be administered into the gluteus medius muscle of the buttock, the vastus lateralis muscle of the thigh or the deltoid muscle of the arm. These sites are used as they reduce the problem of injury to underlying tissues such as nerves and/or major blood vessels (Fig. 1.1).

A subcutaneous injection can be administered in the upper outer aspect of the arm or thigh, the abdomen and the buttock (Fig. 1.2). If a patient is receiving subcutaneous injections over a period of time the site of injection should be rotated to reduce subcutaneous irritation and maintain the medicine absorption rate. Some medicines for subcutaneous injection administration, e.g. insulin or heparin, utilise a prepacked syringe and short needle which requires a similar technique as in intramuscular injection, i.e. needle inserted at a 90° angle.

Communicating

The nurse should help to reinforce any information given to the patient by the medical practitioner about the prescribed medicine and its effect within the patient's body.

Information about a known allergy to a specific medication is usually requested during a patient's admission assessment.

Observation of the effectiveness of a medicine is important, such as following administration of an analgesic. Any sign of the development of a side effect, non-effectiveness or dependence should be reported to the medical practitioner.

Most medications are known to have some form of side effect which can vary between minor upset and a life-threatening event; the nurse should have a knowledge of the side effects of the medicine she is administering. When a side effect is not life threatening it may be necessary for the patient to adjust to a change in his activity of living. The nurse therefore has a role as an educator and facilitator during the adjustment.

Suggested reading

Bird C 1990 Patient self medication. Nursing Times 86(43) October 24: 52–55

Boore J, Champion R, Ferguson M (eds) 1987 Nursing the physically ill adult. Churchill Livingstone, Edinburgh, pp 343–368

Booth S, Booth B 1986 Aperients can be deceptive. Nursing Times 82(39) September 24: 38–39

Burton S 1988 Handling of cytotoxic drugs. Professional Nurse 3(12) September: 496–498

Carlisle D 1990 Nurse prescribing: just what the nurse ordered? Nursing Times 86(29) July 18: 26–28

Freeman E 1990 Making sense of cytotoxic chemotherapy. Nursing Times 86(31) August 1: 45–47

Goodall C 1986 Calculating drug dosages.Nursing Times 82(36) September 3: 44–46

Keen M 1986 Comparison of intramuscular injection technique to reduce site discomfort and lesions. Nursing Research 35(4) July: 207–210

Mathieson A 1986 Old people and drugs. Nursing Times 82(2) January 8: 22–25

Purkiss R, Yuk Chung S 1990 Facing the fax (use of fax machines between the ward and pharmacy). Nursing Times 86(11) March 14: 57–59

Roper N, Logan W, Tierney A 1990 The elements of nursing, 3rd edn. Churchill Livingstone, Edinburgh, p 95

Smith S 1987 Drugs and the heart. Nursing Times 83(21) May 29: 24–26

Smith S 1987 Drugs in angina and myocardial infarction. Nursing Times 83(22) June 3: 52–54

Smith S 1987 Diuretic agents. Nursing Times 83(23) June 10: 53–55

Smith S 1987 Drugs and the parasympathetic nervous system. Nursing Times 83(24) June 17: 36–38

Smith S 1987 Drugs and the gastrointestinal tract. Nursing Times 83(26) July 1: 50–52

Torrance C 1989 Intramuscular injection. Surgical Nurse 2(5) October: 6–10

Torrance C 1989 Intramuscular injection. Surgical Nurse 2(6) December: 24–27

Walsh M, Ford P 1989 Nursing rituals – research and rational actions. Heinemann Nursing, Oxford, ch 8

Williams A 1990 Breaking the chain reaction (common errors in administration). Nursing Times 86(44) October 31: 39–41

Williams A, Winfield A 1990 Topical medications for eye patients. Nursing Times 86(27) July 4: 42–43

Preoperative Nursing Care

Objectives

By the end of this section you should know how to:

- explain the standard preoperative preparations of a patient who is scheduled for surgery

- describe the nurse's role in looking after a patient prior to surgery

Related information

Revision of the cardiopulmonary system.

Review of health authority policy on preoperative preparation of patients.

Guidelines for this nursing practice

- explain the pre- and postoperative routines to the patient and answer any questions appropriately; the discussion of any fears or anxieties that the patient may have should be encouraged

- record the temperature, pulse, respiration, blood pressure and urinalysis to give baseline findings with which to compare postoperative observations

- carry out evacuation of the patient's bowel using suppositories or specific bowel preparation requested by the surgeon

- offer the sedative which will have been ordered by medical staff the night before surgery

- fast the patient for 4–6 hours prior to surgery so that the stomach is empty, in order to avoid the risk of regurgitation and the inhalation of gastric contents while under anaesthesia

- prepare the skin according to health authority policy. This may involve removal of an area of body hair by shaving or depilatory cream; showering or bathing using an antiseptic soap; putting on a theatre gown, and perhaps socks and paper pants

- ensure that all underwear has been removed, although paper pants may be worn on some occasions. Nail varnish should be removed from finger- and toenails so that they can be examined by the anaesthetist for signs of hypoxia, and make-up should be removed for the same reason. Dentures must be removed because of the danger of inhaling them and causing asphyxiation. Health authority policies vary about the removal of spectacles, hairgrips, contact lenses, hearing aids and other prostheses, e.g. wigs, artificial eyes or limbs

- tape the wedding ring to the patient's finger but all other jewellery and valuables which the patient has brought into hospital should be recorded, put into an envelope, appropriately labelled, and placed in a valuables box or safe

- check the patient's identification verbally and from his identiband and confirm that the consent for operation form has been signed

- administer the premedication ordered by the anaesthetist, after the patient has emptied his bladder

- leave the patient to rest quietly when the premedication has been given but observe for reaction to premedication drugs

- when the porter from the theatre reception area arrives to collect the patient, accompany him to the theatre reception area, and hand the patient over to the care of a theatre nurse. There is usually a form with a checklist which the ward nurse and theatre nurse will confirm. The patient may travel to theatre on a hospital bed or on a theatre trolley, according to health authority policy

Relevance to the activities of living

Maintaining a safe environment

Preoperative skin care may vary, as each surgeon has his own theories about any necessary skin preparation to help avoid infection of the wound. Putting clean linen on the bed for the patient's return from theatre is another measure which helps to prevent infection.

It is essential that there is careful identification of the patient to ensure that the patient has the correct operation.

Patient safety while under the influence of premedication is the nurse's responsibility.

It is also the nurse's responsibility to ensure that the patient's valuables are listed and safely stored.

Communicating

Information and explanations are an important part of the nurse's responsibility for patients in surgical wards. Research has shown that explanations prior to surgery can help reduce the incidence of postoperative pain and complications.

A brief description of what to expect in the immediate postoperative period can often be reassuring to the patient, especially if equipment such as urethral catheters, wound drains or intravenous infusion will be in use.

When the patient is being anaesthetised, hearing is the last sense to disappear, so staff should ensure that the content of conversation in the vicinity of the patient will not increase his anxiety.

Breathing

The patient should be encouraged to stop smoking before surgery, to enable the lung fields to be as clear as possible and lessen the susceptibility to pulmonary infection. Breathing exercises should be explained to the patient. These consist of encouraging the patient to sit as upright as possible and to breathe deeply in through his nose, expanding the chest and abdominal wall as much as possible. This allows good inflation of the lungs. On exhaling, the chest and abdominal walls should be allowed to relax and then extra air pushed out of the lungs. The wound can be supported if necessary.

Eating and drinking

As mentioned in the guidelines the patient should be fasted for 4–6 hours prior to surgery to avoid the danger of inhaling gastric contents while the cough reflex is reduced during general anaesthesia. If this has not been possible, e.g. in an emergency admission, it may be necessary to pass a nasogastric tube and aspirate the stomach contents.

Research has shown that prolonged periods of fasting reduce blood glucose levels to below normal range and also cause the patient to become dehydrated. This can impair the healing process and reduce the body's ability to cope with the trauma of surgery.

Relevance to the
activities of living
continued

Eliminating

It is necessary for the patient to have an empty bladder and rectum, especially if muscle relaxant drugs are going to be used during surgery. Otherwise there is the risk of contaminating the theatre table with excrement and the attendant risk of infecting the surgical wound. In addition, in abdominal surgery a full bladder is more liable to be damaged; in emergency surgery, the bladder may be catheterised to obviate this potential complication.

Personal cleansing and dressing

As mentioned in the guidelines, special skin preparation may be required, although some research has shown that the bacterial skin count is less when skin cleansing is done in theatre rather than some hours prior to surgery.

The discussion about removal and method of removal of body hair from around the site of surgery is ongoing and unresolved.

Mobilising

The patient should receive some teaching preoperatively about postoperative exercises to prevent such complications as pressure sores, deep venous thrombosis, chest infections. Nursing staff should ensure that the physiotherapist has visited the patient to give this teaching.

Expressing sexuality

Having to remove all personal clothing, jewellery, make-up, nail varnish and dentures can make the patient feel that personality and personal dignity are threatened. An explanation for these procedures should be given and the assurance that as soon as possible after surgery the patient's wishes regarding cleansing and dressing will be met.

Sleeping

The patient's normal sleeping pattern may be disturbed by the unaccustomed noise of the ward, change of environment, or by anxiety, and every possible means should be used to reduce or remove the cause of anxiety and promote comfort. Medication may be ordered to promote sleep on the night prior to surgery.

Dying

Dying while anaesthetised is not an uncommon fear. The patient should be helped to verbalise and discuss this fear and be helped to realise that with modern technology, such an occurrence is rare.

Many patients facing surgery benefit from attention to their spiritual needs by the hospital chaplain who is a member of the caring team.

Suggested reading

Boore J 1978 Prescription for recovery. Royal College of Nursing, London

Boore J, Champion R, Ferguson M (eds) 1987 Nursing the physically ill adult. Churchill Livingstone, Edinburgh, pp 343–368

Burchill P 1986 Body builders. Nursing Times Community Outlook 82(33) August 13: 19–22 (Discusses the importance of good nutrition for wound healing)

Davis B 1982 Tell them like it is. Nursing Mirror 152(12) March 24: 26–28 (Research study into use of patient information booklets preoperatively and postoperatively)

Hamilton-Smith S 1972 Nil by mouth? Royal College of Nursing, London

Kalideen N 1990 Preparing skin for surgery. Nursing 4(15) September: 28–29

Llewellyn T 1990 Preoperative skin preparation. Surgical Nurse 3(2) April: 24–26

Peters D 1983 Bowel preparation for surgery. Nursing Times 79(28) July 13: 32–34

Roper N, Logan W, Tierney A 1990 The elements of nursing, 3rd edn. Churchill Livingstone, Edinburgh, pp 223–226

Sofaer B 1983 Pain relief – the core of nursing practice. Nursing Times 79(47) November 23: 38–41

Sofaer B 1983 Pain relief – the importance of communication. Nursing Times 79(48) November 30: 32–35

Thomas E 1987 Preoperative fasting – a question of routine? Nursing Times 83(49) December 9: 46–47

Wachstein J 1987 Care of the elderly surgical patient. Geriatric Nursing and Home Care 7(4) April: 12–14

Winfield U 1986 Too close a shave? Nursing Times 82(10) March 10: 64, 67–68

Postoperative Nursing Care

Objectives

By the end of this section you should know how to:

- explain the general postoperative care of a patient
- describe the nurse's role in carrying out general postoperative care

Related information

Revision of the clinical features of shock.

Revision of the physiology of wound healing.

Review of health authority policy about postoperative care.

Guidelines for this nursing practice

When receiving the patient back into the ward:

- check that the airway is patent and that the patient is breathing adequately. Usually the patient is conscious before leaving the recovery room
- record the temperature, pulse and blood pressure and compare the results with the patient's preoperative recordings
- observe the wound and any drains which may be present, e.g. Redivac, catheter
- check, if an intravenous infusion is present, that it is functioning according to medical staff instructions

- read the patient's theatre notes to confirm the surgical procedure which has been carried out and ascertain any instructions from the surgeon or anaesthetist, e.g. positioning of the patient, oxygen therapy
- ensure that the patient is lying in as comfortable a position as possible, and that the limbs are positioned in a manner which will not endanger muscle and nerve tissue
- administer analgesia as required by the patient and as prescribed by the medical staff

Continuing postoperative nursing:

- record blood pressure, pulse and respiration rates until they are within normal range and stable
- assist the patient to wash and change into his own nightwear and offer a mouthwash
- encourage the patient to sit up in bed well supported by pillows (unless contraindicated) and move around as much as able, helping him out of bed when blood pressure recordings are satisfactory
- allow graduated amounts of fluid unless contraindicated (e.g. the presence of a nasogastric tube), then gradually introduce solid food if there is no vomiting and if bowel sounds are present

- record the amount and time when the patient passes urine and when he has a first bowel movement
- ensure that the patient has adequate periods of rest
- give encouragement and support to the patient and any explanation or information he may require
- the breathing exercises described in the appropriate section on p. 19 should be encouraged

Relevance to the activities of living

Maintaining a safe environment

All precautions must be taken for prevention of infection, e.g. a strict aseptic technique should be used when carrying out wound care. An appropriate wound dressing which will promote an ideal healing environment should be prescribed.

While the patient is under the influence of anaesthesia and analgesia his safety is of prime importance and is a nursing responsibility.

Communicating

Hearing is one of the first senses to return after anaesthesia.

Adequate explanations, support and encouragement must be available to the patient at all times. Patient education about surgery and its after-effects must be well planned and carried out by an appropriately qualified member of staff, preferably prior to surgery and reinforced in the postoperative period.

Breathing

Chest infections and pulmonary embolism are potential problems for patients undergoing surgery so patient education prior to surgery about suitable exercises and deep breathing can help to prevent these complications.

The complication of haemorrhage should be detected by monitoring the wound, pulse, blood pressure and the patient's colour.

Eating and drinking

Fluids should be limited to 3 litres for the first 24 hours after surgery because of the excess production of antidiuretic hormone as a result of surgery but thereafter, unless contraindicated, fluid intake should be encouraged.

A gradual return to a normal diet, high in protein and vitamins, should be encouraged, to promote wound healing.

Antiemetics may be prescribed if the patient is suffering from nausea and vomiting.

Eliminating

Anaesthesia can alter bladder muscle tone and may cause difficulty in micturition. It has been demonstrated that anaesthesia can lead to excess secretion of antidiuretic hormone and it can take 24–48 hours for renal function to return to normal. If the patient's bladder becomes very distended, catheterisation may be necessary, although all other activities to encourage micturition are encouraged first.

If the surgery has involved handling the intestines, abdominal distension caused by large amounts of flatus can result causing extreme discomfort. Sometimes a paralytic ileus can develop; the clinical features are abdominal distension, vomiting and absence of bowel sounds and must be reported immediately.

As with the bladder muscle, some forms of anaesthesia can have an effect on the muscle layer of the bowel, and it can take 24–48 hours to return to normal. If the patient has not had a bowel movement by the 3rd postoperative day, a bulk-forming laxative or evacuant suppositories may be administered.

Relevance to the
activities of living
continued

Personal cleansing and dressing

Adequate assistance should be given in the immediate postoperative period but the patient should be encouraged to be independent as soon as possible.

The appearance of the skin over the pressure areas should be observed, and the appearance of the skin around the wound site.

Mobilising

Preoperatively the patient should have been taught about the importance of movement in bed to prevent pressure sores and the development of deep venous thrombosis. The rate of mobilisation will vary depending on the type of surgery carried out, the general condition of the patient, and his personal response to the stress of surgery. A nursing assessment should enable the nurse and patient to plan the most suitable programme of mobilisation for that individual.

Working and playing

Surgery may affect the patient's ability to return to his former employment or hobbies and sport. He should be encouraged and supported while trying to find alternatives.

Expressing sexuality

If surgery results in an altered body image the patient may require support and encouragement to adjust to and accept the change.

Sleeping

The patient's normal sleeping pattern may be altered after surgery due to observations being carried out or because of pain, anxiety, discomfort, noise and connection to unusual equipment. Medication to induce sleep may be prescribed but only after other measures have been used, e.g. helping the patient to find a more comfortable position, relieving pain, giving a hot, soothing drink, listening to his concerns.

Suggested reading   Boore J 1978 Prescription for recovery. Royal College of Nursing, London
Boore J, Champion R, Ferguson M (eds) 1987 Nursing the physically ill adult. Churchill
     Livingstone, Edinburgh, chs 9, 10, 17
Burchill P 1986 Body builders. Nursing Times Community Outlook 82(33) August 13:
     19–22 (Discusses the importance of good nutrition for wound healing)
Davis B 1982 Tell them like it is. Nursing Mirror 154(12) March 24: 26–28 (Research
     study into the use of patient information booklets preoperatively and postoperatively)
Roper N, Logan W, Tierney A 1990 The elements of nursing, 3rd edn. Churchill
     Livingstone, Edinburgh, pp 121–125
Sofaer B 1983 Pain relief – the core of nursing practice. Nursing Times 79(47)
     November 23: 38–41
Sofaer B 1983 Pain relief – the importance of communication. Nursing Times 79(48)
     December 7: 32–35
Wachstein J 1987 Care of the elderly surgical patient. Geriatric Nursing and Home
     Care 7(4) April: 12–14

Aseptic Technique

There are three parts to this section:

1 Aseptic wound dressing
2 Wound drain care
3 Removal of stitches, clips or staples

The concluding subsection, 'Relevance to the activities of living', refers to the three practices collectively.

Objectives

By the end of this section you should know how to:

- prepare the patient for these three nursing practices
- collect and prepare the equipment
- carry out these nursing practices

Related information

Revision of wound classification.

Revision of the physiology of wound healing and the factors which affect wound healing.

Review of the health authority policies regarding all three parts of aseptic technique.

1 ASEPTIC WOUND DRESSING

Some indications for an aseptic wound dressing

This is the technique used to reduce the potential problem of introducing pathogenic microorganisms into the body when the integrity and/or effectiveness of the natural body defences has been reduced. The details of the technique may be modified according to the particular dressings pack which is used, but the principles are the same. The equipment, lotions and dressings used are sterile and the risk of contamination by airborne pathogenic microorganisms is kept to a minimum. Aseptic wound dressing can be indicated:

- following surgery when skin continuity has been interrupted
- following trauma to the skin tissue
- during an invasive procedure such as catheterisation or introduction of an intravenous cannula

Equipment

Dressings trolley
Sterile dressings pack containing a gallipot or similar container, cotton wool balls, gauze swabs, disposable forceps and drape
Sterile wound-cleansing lotion e.g. normal saline
Additional sterile dressing material, usually packed separately
Hypoallergenic tape
Clean pair of scissors for cutting tape
Clean disposable plastic apron
Alcohol-based hand preparation lotion
Receptacle for soiled disposables

Guidelines for this nursing practice

- explain the nursing practice to the patient and gain his consent and cooperation
- if a treatment room is not available for wound dressing technique, prepare the environment around the patient's bed
- wash the hands
- wash the dressings trolley thoroughly with detergent and water and then dry
- disinfect the dressings trolley with 70% ethyl alcohol immediately prior to every dressing technique
- collect and prepare the equipment by checking all packaging for damage such as tears or leakage. Check the expiry dates of all the equipment
- place all the equipment on the bottom shelf of the trolley preferably in the order of use
- attach receptacle for soiled disposables to the side of the trolley below the level of the top shelf. This assists in reducing contamination from the soiled disposables to the top shelf of the dressing trolley during the dressing
- ensure the patient's privacy
- observe the patient throughout this activity
- help the patient into a comfortable position
- adjust the patient's clothing to expose the wound area
- wash the hands
- apply the plastic disposable apron
- open the outer packaging of the dressings pack and slip onto the top shelf of the dressings trolley
- loosen the outer dressing covering the patient's wound

- wash the hands using the alcohol-based hand lotion
- open the dressings pack touching the sterile covering as little as possible to reduce contamination by the dresser's hands
- using one pair of forceps from the contents of the dressings pack arrange the equipment on the sterile field
- open additional equipment and drop onto the sterile field. Pour skin cleansing lotion into the gallipot
- using forceps remove the soiled dressing and discard both the dressing and forceps
- drape the wound with the sterile drape if used
- note the condition of the wound and surrounding tissue
- if used, apply sterile disposable gloves which can be used instead of forceps for the swabbing of the wound
- cleanse the wound using one swab once only, working from the centre of the wound outwards and from the cleanest part first. These measures may reduce the danger of cross-infection
- apply the new dressing
- discard gloves or forceps
- secure the dressing
- ensure that the patient is left feeling as comfortable as possible
- dispose of all equipment safely
- document this nursing practice appropriately, monitor after-effects and report abnormal findings immediately

2 WOUND DRAIN CARE

Some indications for wound drain care

Wound drains are inserted at the time of surgical intervention by the medical practitioner to prevent fluid collecting at the operation or wound site, a factor which may retard tissue healing. The extent and site of the surgery will influence the type and number of drains used. Drains may be inserted away from the original incision to be dressed and heal independently. They are frequently stitched in position and attached to a closed circuit drainage bag, or portable suction if required.

Some types of wound drains

Hollow plastic tube: this is a deep drain with drainage holes at the proximal (drainage site) end. It is usually stitched in position and attached to a closed circuit drainage bag. It may be used following major abdominal surgery.

Corrugated rubber drain: this is a superficial drain which usually drains directly into the dressing. It may be used to drain an incision site.

T-tube: this is a specialised tube inserted into the common bile duct following a cholecystectomy. It allows bile to drain into a closed circuit bag for 6–10 days postoperatively, until normal drainage is re-established.

Portable vacuum suction drain: this is a perforated plastic catheter attached to a specialised sterile vacuum suction bag. Two or more may be attached to the same vacuum bag with a Y connection. This system is used to prevent a haematoma forming by maintaining gentle suction. It may be used following joint replacement surgery (Fig. 1.3) or surgery in the face or neck area.

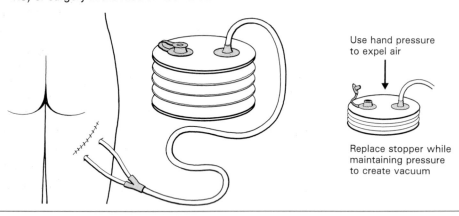

Figure 1.3
Wound care: a portable vacuum drain

Use hand pressure to expel air

Replace stopper while maintaining pressure to create vacuum

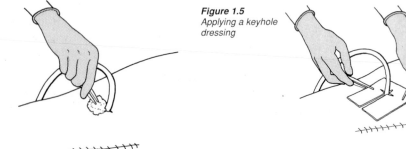

Figure 1.4
Cleansing the skin round the wound drain

Figure 1.5
Applying a keyhole dressing

Equipment   As for aseptic wound dressing (see Aseptic technique p. 26)

Additional equipment as required

Sterile gloves
Sterile scissors
Sterile stitch cutters
Sterile drainage bag
Portable wound suction equipment
Sterile specialised keyhole dressing
Extra sterile dressings material
Sterile safety pin
Sterile wound pads
Measuring jug
Sterile specimen container

Sterile gloves should be used when dressing wound drains to help maintain asepsis and to protect nursing staff from any infected body fluids

Guidelines for this nursing practice

- explain the nursing practice to the patient and gain his consent and cooperation

- ensure the patient's privacy

- help the patient into a comfortable position depending on the area of the wound drain

- observe the patient throughout this activity

- collect and prepare the equipment

- remove clothes and covers from the area of the wound ensuring that apart from that area, the patient remains covered

- perform the dressing for the surgical incision line first if necessary, maintaining asepsis. Normally dressings will be removed from the incision line after 24 hours, and the wound covered by plastic spray dressing. After this only the drainage tube sites need to be dressed

- prepare the sterile field for dressing the drainage tube site

- don sterile gloves

- proceed as for aseptic technique until the drainage tube is exposed

- cleanse the skin round the wound drain with wound cleansing lotion (Fig. 1.4)

- dry the skin round the wound drain

- prepare a 'keyhole dressing'. This allows the dressing to fit snugly round the drain (Fig. 1.5)

- shorten the drain as ordered by the medical practitioner

- apply the keyhole dressing or other as required

- secure the dressing

- change the drainage bag and secure it in position

- measure the drainage fluid and note its colour, consistency and smell

- ensure that the patient is left as comfortable as possible

- dispose of the equipment safely

- document this nursing practice appropriately, monitor after-effects and report abnormal findings immediately

Guidelines for this
nursing practice
continued

Shortening wound drains

Deep wound drains may be shortened once or twice during the postoperative period as healing proceeds, as ordered by the medical practitioner:

- expose the drain site maintaining asepsis, cleansing the skin as before. Sterile gloves should be worn

- remove any stitches holding the drain in position (see removal of stitches p. 31)

- support the skin round the drain site with one hand using a sterile s ab and gently withdraw the drain as far as ordered by the medical practitioner, e.g. 3–5 cm

- insert a sterile safety pin through the drain near the entry site. This prevents the drain falling back into the wound

- cut off the extra length of drain if necessary. Drains attached to drainage bags will not need to be cut

- apply a sterile keyhole dressing under the safety pin, and another over the safety pin. This helps to maintain the drain in position, and prevents the safety pin from damaging the skin

- secure the dressing in position

- proceed as for 'Guidelines for this nursing practice'

Removing wound drains

This will be ordered by the medical practitioner when there is no longer any significant drainage from the wound:

- expose the drain site, cleanse the skin as before, maintaining asepsis. Sterile gloves should be worn

- remove any stitches holding the drain in position

- support the skin round the drain site with one hand, using a sterile swab, and gently withdraw the drain using either a sterile gloved hand or sterile forceps held in the other hand. If required for microbiological investigation, the tip of the drain should

be cut off with sterile scissors and placed in a sterile specimen container, maintaining asepsis

- cleanse and dry the wound site again if necessary

- apply and secure an appropriate sterile dressing

- proceed as for 'Guidelines for this nursing practice'

- dispatch the labelled specimen to the laboratory immediately with the form

Emptying the portable wound suction container

The containers should be emptied as soon as they are no longer maintaining a vacuum suction, or every 12 hours as required:

- clamp the drainage tubing above the level of the wound drainage container

- remove the stopper or bung from the container, maintaining asepsis

- obtain a specimen of drainage fluid for microbiological investigation if required

- pour the remaining contents into a measuring jug

- wipe the outside of the entry channel with alcohol solution, e.g. Mediswab

- press the two rigid surfaces of the container together and maintain the pressure until the stopper is firmly in position. Once the pressure is removed a gentle vacuum suction is created

- secure the drainage bag in position

- document the amount and details of the drainage fluid in the patient's records

3   REMOVAL OF STITCHES, CLIPS OR STAPLES

Some indications for removal of stitches, clips or staples

Following surgery, stitches, clips or staples are used to place the skin edges in apposition and promote rapid healing. These are removed when there is:

- evidence of the wound having healed
- infection in part of the wound

Equipment

Sterile dressings pack
Water-based antiseptic for wound cleansing
Sterile stitch cutter or scissors, clip or staple remover
Receptacle for soiled disposables

Guidelines for this nursing practice

Figure 1.6
Removal of sutures, clips and staples

- explain the procedure to the patient to gain his consent and cooperation
- ensure the patient's privacy
- collect the equipment

- observe the patient throughout this activity
- clean the wound with antiseptic only if it is necessary to get access to stitches, clips or staples

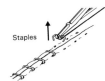

Sutures

Removing sutures

- hold the stitch cutter or scissors in the dominant hand and the dissecting forceps in the other hand to lift gently the knot of the stitch (Fig. 1.6)
- cut between the knot and the skin, so that no part of the stitch above the skin surface is pulled under the tissues, then gently pull out the cut stitch

- ensure that no piece of the stitch is left in the wound, as this could eventually form a wound sinus

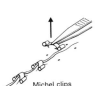

Staples

Removing clips or staples

- hold the remover in the dominant hand and the dissecting forceps in the other hand when removing clips or staples (Fig. 1.6)
- steady the clips or staples with the dissecting forceps. Depending on the type of clip or staple, either insert one blade of the remover under the centre of the clip or staple and the other blade over, then gently squeeze blades together OR place a blade of the remover on the outside of each wing on top of the clip and squeeze the blades together. Depending on the clip or staple type, one or other of these actions should lift the clip from the skin on either side of the wound

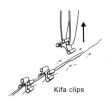

Michel clips

Kifa clips

- follow health authority policy for the aftercare of a wound. The wound may be cleaned if necessary then left exposed, covered with a dry sterile dressing or sprayed with a waterproof plastic film
- ensure the patient is left as comfortable as possible
- dispose of all equipment safely
- document the nursing practice appropriately, monitor after-effects and report abnormal findings immediately

Aseptic Technique

Relevance to the activities of living

Maintaining a safe environment

In a healthy individual the skin and mucous membranes act as a natural defence against the entry of pathogenic microorganisms. When continuity of these tissues is lost even temporarily, there is the potential for creating infection. Infection of any kind is an extremely debilitating process. It can cause a great deal of discomfort and inconvenience to the patient, as well as increasing the length of stay in hospital and hospital costs.

Airborne pathogenic microorganisms can be reduced by utilising a well ventilated room solely used for procedures involving aseptic technique, or by performing procedures at least 30 minutes after completion of ward cleaning and bedmaking. This may not always be possible.

There is no need for the nurse to wear a disposable cap or face mask but verbal communication should be kept to a minimum during the aseptic technique, to reduce droplet contamination. When a number of aseptic wound dressings are to be performed, a known contaminated and/or infected wound should be left to the last to reduce the environmental contamination.

Careful preparation of the equipment to be used can further reduce environmental contamination. The dressings trolley should be washed using detergent and water then dried on a daily basis, and immediately prior to the preparation for aseptic technique it should be disinfected with 70% ethyl alcohol. It is preferable that the dressings trolley be solely used for that purpose. All equipment packaging should be checked for damage and date of expiry which would render the equipment non-sterile.

The member of staff who performs aseptic technique also requires specific preparation. Due to the nature of the nurse's work her uniform and hands can be a catchment area for pathogenic microorganisms. A disposable plastic apron should be worn to provide a barrier to transmission of microorganisms. Thorough hand washing *prior* to the trolley preparation, using preferably an antiseptic detergent wash, must be performed. Further hand preparation should be performed *during* the aseptic technique as stated in the guidelines, and when the nurse accidentally contaminates her hands. Alcohol-based hand rub is being used for the subsequent hand preparation; it has the benefit that the nurse does not have to leave the patient's bedside during the practice.

It is preferable that the skin cleansing lotion be supplied as an individual single-use sterile sachet or bottle. Once a bottle has been opened environmental contamination can occur, therefore the residual lotion following aseptic technique should be discarded.

Continual use of aseptic skin cleansing lotion may have a detrimental effect on granulation tissue. Adequate wound cleansing of an open granulating wound can be achieved with the use of sterile normal saline.

A non-touch technique reduces the potential problem of contamination from the nurse's hands to the wound. Sterile forceps or gloves can be used, the latter having the benefit of easing manipulative skills. As the soiled dressing and equipment used during removal may be contaminated, all items must be discarded before continuing with the aseptic technique. The wound should be cleansed and dried thoroughly using each swab once only, working from the centre of the wound outwards and from the cleanest part first. These measures may reduce cross-infection from one part of the wound to another.

On completion of the aseptic technique discard all equipment in the appropriate receptacles and seal them, before leaving the patient, to reduce environmental contamination from the soiled equipment. The trolley should be washed, dried and returned to its place of storage. The nurse should thoroughly wash her hands using soap and water only.

As a wound drain is in direct contact with the underlying tissues, pathogenic microorganisms could gain entry to a wound through the drain site. Maintenance of a closed drainage system and aseptic technique may help to reduce the chance of wound infection.

A wound drain site should be dressed after the incision site to minimise the risk of cross-infection. Gauze swabs should not be cut for keyhole dressings as small pieces of cut gauze may remain within the wound. Commercial keyhole dressings are available with sealed edges. If unavailable any suitable sterile dressing may be placed around the drain and secured in position to cover the drain site.

During suture, clip or staple removal, care must be taken to prevent the sharp equipment causing accidental injury to the patient.

Communicating

The nursing practice should be explained simply to the patient. Any discomfort or pain should be anticipated by the nurse and the appropriate analgesic offered, as prescribed by a medical practitioner.

The nurse should inform the patient of her intended actions during the nursing practice as this may help to reduce his anxiety.

An explanation for reduced verbal communication during aseptic technique should be given. The nurse must be alert to the fact that her non-verbal communication can often be interpreted by a patient, e.g. when faced with a malodorous or unsightly wound a reaction of disgust must not be evident. Observation of the patient's non-verbal communication may be an indicator of his acceptance of a change in his body image if the wound is defacing.

The nurse should observe and note any sign of inflammation such as increased heat, redness or swelling around the wound as this may indicate the presence of infection.

Breathing

The patient's respiration and pulse rates may increase due to anxiety.

Eliminating

The patient should empty his bladder prior to these nursing interventions to facilitate comfort.

Personal cleansing and dressing

Care must be taken during the performance of this activity of living that the wound dressing or drain comes to no harm.

In some hospital departments, surgical wounds are left exposed to the environment within the first few days of surgery. If this is practised the dried blood along the suture line should not be removed because this acts as a protective barrier.

Relevance to the
activities of living
continued

When securing a dressing with tape allow for body movement when applying it, i.e. stretch out any natural skin creases during the application. Wet wound dressings should be changed immediately except during the first 24 hours following surgery, when the dressing is used as an estimation of approximate fluid loss.

Even before the removal of sutures, clips or staples, an immersion bath or shower can usually be performed by the patient with assistance from the nurse, but this will vary within hospitals and departments.

Following removal of sutures, clips and staples, advice may have to be given to the patient about aftercare of a healing wound and the most appropriate clothing to wear. The area should be washed and dried carefully each day. The clothing worn on top of the wound should not be tight but may be gently supportive if desired.

Wound dressing deodorants may be found to be useful in concealing the smell from a malodorous wound.

Controlling body temperature

A patient with an infected wound may develop pyrexia. The nurse should implement the appropriate nursing intervention to assist the patient if this complication occurs.

Mobilising

A wound dressing should not impede mobilising, but due to discomfort, the presence of a wound drain, or awkwardness of the site of the wound, may interfere with the patient's normal form of mobilising.

A patient may fear that the sutures, clips or staples holding the wound may give way when mobilising. The nurse should allay his fears and explain the importance and benefit of adequate mobilisation.

The patient may fear that the wound will open up following removal of the wound closures. Some education and guidance may be necessary and many surgical units have printed leaflets with advice and information which can be given to the patient to read at leisure.

Expressing sexuality

Adequate provision of privacy is essential in reducing patient anxiety during these interventions. The nurse should assist the patient in adjusting to any altered body image whether the disfigurement is temporary or permanent.

Sleeping

The patient's normal sleep pattern may be altered due to the discomfort caused by the presence of a wound dressing and drain. The appropriate nursing intervention may be helping the patient to find a more comfortable position or it may be listening to his concerns and helping him to allay anxiety or it may be administering a prescribed analgesic to reduce discomfort and pain.

Suggested reading *Aseptic technique*

Alexander J, O'Connor H 1982 The Hampshire dressing aid. Nursing 2(8) December, Supplement: 6–7

Ayton M 1987 A healing process. Senior Nurse 6(4) ·April: 21–23

Cubby C 1990 Which dressing? Nursing Times 86(15) April 11: 63–64

Dealey C 1989 Management of cavity wounds. Nursing 3(39) July: 25–27

Fincham Gee C 1990 Nutrition and wound healing. Nursing 4(18) September 13: 26–28

Gilchrist B 1990 Washing and dressings after surgery. Nursing Times 86(50) December 12: 71

Hill S 1984 Which disinfectants do nurses use? Nursing Times 80(7) February 15: 60–61

Irvine A, Black C 1990 Pressure sore practices (discusses wound dressings). Nursing Times 86(38) September 19: 74–78

Kelso H 1989 Alternative technique. Nursing Times 85(23) June 7: 40–42

Larson E 1985 Evaluating handwashing techniques. Journal of Advanced Nursing 10(6) December: 547–552

O'Brien 1986 Postoperative wound infections. Nursing 3(5) May: 178–182

Roper N, Logan W, Tierney A 1990 The elements of nursing, 3rd edn. Churchill Livingstone, Edinburgh, pp 74–83, 92–95

Spanswick A, Gibbs S, Ekeland P 1990 Eusol – the final word! Professional Nurse 5(4) January: 211–212

Sutton J 1989 Accurate wound assessment. Nursing Times 85(38) September 20: 68–71

Taylor L 1978 An evaluation of handwashing techniques – 1. Nursing Times 74(2) January 12: 54–55

Taylor L 1978 An evaluation of handwashing techniques – 2. Nursing Times 74(3) January 19: 108–110

Thomas S 1990 Making sense of hydrocolloid dressings. Nursing Times 86(4) November 7: 36–38

Walsh M, Ford P 1989 Nursing rituals – research and rational actions. Heinemann Nursing, Oxford, Ch 2

Westaby S 1985 Wound care. Heinemann, London, pp 32–46

Wound drain care

Davis B, Blenkharn I 1987 On the right track. Nursing Times, Journal of Infection Control Nursing 83(22) June 3: 64–68 (Discusses the hazards of suction apparatus)

Kalideen D 1990 Preparing skin for surgery. Nursing 4(15) July 26: 28–29

Molyneux R 1983 A preliminary investigation into surgical dressings used over postoperative passive wound drains. Journal of Advanced Nursing 8(6) November: 525–533

Nightingale K 1989 Making sense of wound drainage. Nursing Times 85(27) July 5: 40–42

Walsh M, Ford P 1989 Nursing rituals, research and rational actions. Heinemann Nursing, Oxford, pp 22–27

Wound sutures, clips and staples

Nightingale K 1990 Making sense of wound closure. Nursing Times 86(14) April 4: 35–37

Poole D 1982 Suturing techniques. Nursing 2(11) March: 306–307

Isolation Nursing

There are three parts to this section:

1 **Source isolation**
2 **Protective isolation**
3 **Radioactive hazard isolation**

The concluding subsection, 'Relevance to the activities of living', refers to the three practices collectively.

Objectives

By the end of this section you should know how to:

- prevent the spread of infection while nursing a patient with a specific communicable disease (source isolation)

- protect a patient from infection when he may be at a greater risk than normal (protective isolation)

- prevent hazard to carers and visitors when radioactive substances are used

Related information

Revision of the modes of transmission of infection and related microbiology.

Review of health authority policy in relation to control of infection.

Review of health authority policy in relation to the handling of radioactive substances.

Some indications for isolation nursing

The aim of this nursing practice is to create an effective barrier between an infected area and a non-infected area, or to use appropriate measures to prevent contamination from radioactive substances.

1   SOURCE ISOLATION (BARRIER NURSING)

In this instance the infected area is the isolation area where the infected patient is nursed, and the non-infected area is outside the isolation area.

Some indications for source isolation

This is carried out to prevent the spread of infection *from*:

- patients who have or are suspected of having a specific communicable infection, for example:
  — a wound infection caused by *Staphylococcus aureus*
  — a respiratory infection caused by tuberculosis
  — an enteric infection caused by salmonella

Equipment

Equipment will depend on the infection, the patient's condition and health authority policies.

Single room with toilet facilities

Hand washing facilities for personnel inside and outside the isolation area

Alcohol solution for rinsing hands

Protective clothing, which may include:
— cap
— filter-type mask
— gown
— plastic apron
— gloves
— overshoes
— goggles

These should be disposable and a supply kept just outside the isolation area

Disposable or individual crockery and cutlery

Facilities for treatment of, or disposal of, infected linen and rubbish

All equipment needed for appropriate nursing care should remain within the isolation area. The area should be equipped with a thermometer, sphygmomanometer, stethoscope and a watch or clock with a seconds hand as required for recording vital signs.

The patient's documentation should remain outside the isolation area and details of recordings and care completed by 'uncontaminated' personnel.

Guidelines for this nursing practice

- consult appropriate personnel for advice and guidance. Most health authorities and hospitals have a member of staff designated to be responsible for the control of infection in that area

- plan the nursing so that everything required is carried out during one period of time in the isolation area. Personnel continually entering and leaving the area greatly increase the risk of cross-infection

- choose personnel with known immunity to care for patients with specific infections if possible

- explain the importance of the precautions to the patient and gain his consent and cooperation

- wash hands and apply alcohol solution before entering the isolation area

- don protective clothing as required

- enter the isolation area

- perform all necessary nursing. Two nurses may be needed for certain nursing practices, e.g. to pass in any equipment, the patient's meals, or prescribed medication from outside the isolation area. One nurse should remain in protective clothing within the area. The second nurse should remain at the entrance of the area and transfer articles to the nurse within the area without allowing any contamination to occur

- observe the patient throughout this activity

- ensure that the patient is left feeling as comfortable as possible

- ensure that the patient has a means of communication, e.g. bell, two-way radio

- safely dispose of any infected material according to health authority policies

- wash hands within the isolation area

- remove protective clothing without touching the ouside of the garments and dispose of it

- leave the isolation area

- repeat hand washing outside the isolation area and apply alcohol solution

- document the nursing practices appropriately, monitor after-effects and report abnormal findings immediately

- explain the precautions to visitors, who should be restricted to close relatives and friends and obtain their cooperation in maintaining isolation for the patient by wearing protective clothing

Disposal of infected material

Two nurses are required; one to remain in her protective clothing within the isolation area, the second nurse to remain free from contamination outside the isolation area.

Disposal of waste: This should be put in a clinical waste disposal bag and closed as appropriate inside the isolation area by the isolation nurse. The second nurse from outside the area remains at the entrance with an open clinical waste bag into which the isolation nurse places the infected bag without touching the outside of the second bag. The second bag is closed without contaminating the outside, and treated as normal clinical waste. This procedure is known as 'double bagging' (Fig. 1.7).

Disposal of linen: Infected linen should be 'double bagged' in clear plastic bags and sent to the laundry in carriers designated for infected linen; sometimes disposable linen is used.

Disposal of sharps: The infected sharps container should be safely closed by the isolation nurse and placed in a clear plastic bag held by the second nurse, keeping the outside uncontaminated.

Domestic cleaning

The domestic manager should be informed whenever isolation procedures are required. Arrangements for cleaning the isolation area will be made in cooperation with the hospital infection control personnel.

Decontamination of the isolation area

When a patient leaves an isolation area, the nursing staff should dispose of all the infected equipment. The room or cubicle and associated furniture should be decontaminated as health authority policy dictates, before being used again.

Specific precautions

Different precautions may be needed for specific infections.

Respiratory infections: The patient should be nursed in a single room or cubicle with the door kept closed to reduce airborne infection.

Masks which act as an efficient barrier should be worn by all personnel entering the area to protect staff from infection.

Gloves should be worn when handling sputum or contaminated linen, and when assisting the patient with oral hygiene. Good hand washing technique should give adequate protection otherwise.

Individual or disposable crockery and cutlery should be used as required.

Urine and faeces do not require special treatment, but the use of a separate toilet or commode helps to reduce cross-infection.

Wound infections: The patient should be nursed in a single room or cubicle.

Gloves should be worn, especially when performing dressings or handling potentially infected bed linen or clothing.

A mask may only be necessary when performing dressings.

A plastic apron may be adequate protective clothing depending on the organism causing the infection.

Good hand washing technique is essential.

Figure 1.7
Isolation nursing; removal of a disposal bag from the infected area to the 'clean' area. Infected bag already tied up is placed inside clean bag held by another nurse outside the area, and tied up without contaminating the outside

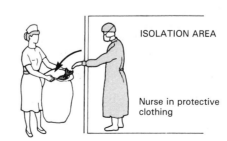

'Clean' nurse

ISOLATION AREA

Nurse in protective clothing

Isolation Nursing

Guidelines for this
nursing practice
continued

Enteric infections: The patient should be nursed in a single room or cubicle with adequate individual toilet facilities.

Gowns, plastic aprons and gloves should be worn, but a mask is not necessary.

Individual or disposable crockery and cutlery should be used as required.

Vomitus and faeces will be infected and should be disposed of according to local policies. This may include covering the infected matter with disinfectant for a period of time.

Toilet utensils should be disposable and treated as infected waste.

Before removing protective clothing, the gloved hands should be washed to reduce contamination and further hand washing performed as in the Guidelines given above.

Viral infections: Special precautions are applicable when a patient has a viral infection caused by:
— Hepatitis B virus
— Human immunodeficiency virus (HIV) which may develop into acquired immune deficiency syndrome (AIDS)

These patients may be suffering from the disease or carry the virus in their blood and should be treated as having infected blood and body fluids. The caring personnel are most at risk of infection in this situation. Precautions should be maintained for all patients suspected of being 'carriers' until investigations prove negative. According to current knowledge, the people most likely to be infected are:
— addicts who take drugs by the intravenous route and use contaminated needles
— male homosexuals, especially those with numerous partners
— babies born to mothers who are infected
— people who have been transfused with contaminated blood, or blood products
— patients from, or who have recently visited, tropical or subtropical countries where there is a relatively higher incidence of the disease

Every precaution should be taken to prevent personnel in contact with the patient from being infected by the virus; it would have to enter the blood circulation through a break in the skin or through the mucosa of the non-infected individual. The degree of risk is assessed by the medical practitioner and precautions prescribed accordingly.

Low risk situations: Precautions should be taken when handling blood and body secretions. Gloves should be worn at all times. Special care should be taken when handling and disposing of syringes and needles. Sharps containers should be treated as infected and labelled with special stickers. Blood and other specimens for investigation should be labelled with special stickers and placed in 2 bags before being sent to the laboratory.

High risk situations: Additional precautions may be prescribed, for example when carrying out an invasive procedure for patients known to be infected by HIV or hepatitis B. Strict isolation nursing should be maintained and protective clothing should include goggles worn by attending personnel, as well as efficient masks to prevent any infected secretion or blood splashing the eyes or mouth of the carer. In some areas where such patients are known to be admitted, a protective 'pack' is available for immediate use. The infection control personnel should be the resource centre for any special requirements (refer to health authority policies).

2   PROTECTIVE ISOLATION (REVERSE BARRIER NURSING)

In this situation the infected area is the environment of the ward and the non-infected area is the isolation area. Pathogens are prevented from entering the isolation area by protective isolation for the patient. The principles and the guidelines are the same but the procedure is reversed.

Some indications for protective isolation

This is carried out to prevent the spread of infection to:

- patients who have a reduced resistance to infection due to their disease condition or to prescribed treatment, for example:
  — patients who have leukaemia
  — patients who have reduced autoimmunity due to cytotoxic medication for treatment of malignant disease
  — patients who are receiving immunosuppressive medication following transplant surgery

The following precautions are emphasised:

A filter-type mask must be used by all personnel to protect the patient from any droplet infection.

The form of protective clothing depends on the patient's condition. Gowns should be worn when nursing children, or patients who are at particular risk of infection, but in some instances a plastic apron will be sufficient to prevent any cross-infection from the nurse's uniform.

A cap and overshoes may be worn.

All personnel must be meticulous in their hand washing technique.

Alcohol hand rub should be applied frequently to the nurse's hands to further reduce the risk of cross-infection.

Special air flow facilities, e.g. laminar flow system, may be used to prevent a flow of air from the ward area to the isolation area. This decreases the risk of cross-infection from the ward environment.

The precautions should be explained to the visitors, who should be limited to close relatives and friends, and appropriate protective clothing should be worn.

Visitors and other personnel should not be in contact with the patient if they have a cold, sore throat, or other infection however mild, and the reason for this precaution should be explained.

Nursing should be planned so that only one or two of the staff are caring for the patient during a span of duty to reduce the risk of infection from ward personnel.

3 RADIOACTIVE HAZARD ISOLATION

Patients receiving large doses of radioactive isotopes, either systemically or by implant, are normally nursed in specially equipped units. However, radioactive isotopes are being used more frequently for diagnostic purposes, and nurses may care for patients undergoing such investigations in general wards.

Some indications for radioactive hazard isolation

This is carried out to prevent radioactive contamination to carers and others when radioactive substances are used:

- to treat patients who have malignant tumours with radioactive implants or radioactive isotopes

- for diagnostic investigations using radioactive isotopes

The isolation technique is aimed at reducing the risk of radiation for other patients and caring personnel by limiting the time spent near the patient having radioactive treatment, and keeping a safe distance away at other times. The patient should be nursed in a single room, or confined to one particular area of the ward. Lead screens should be used as a shield from radiation when radioactive implants are inserted, according to individual requirements. Radioactive material should be transported in lead containers.

Guidelines for this nursing practice

- consult the radiation protection officer and health authority policy about appropriate precautions for particular radioactive substances used for treatment or investigations

- explain the precautions and their implications to the patient and gain his consent and cooperation

- ensure that all staff wear radiation detection badges. This will monitor individual doses of radiation and ensure that no one is exposed to dangerous levels

- plan nursing so that no nurse is in an area of radiation for longer than necessary, and share care so that each nurse has a reduced exposure time

- don protective lead aprons if appropriate

- wear gloves for all nursing practices and when handling any bedclothes or linen which may be contaminated by radioactive excreta and body fluid

- dispose of linen and waste according to health authority policy, labelling materials with special radioactive warning stickers

- wear gloves to wipe up any spillages of suspected radioactive material immediately with paper tissues and rinse the area with water. The tissues should be treated as radioactive waste

- dilute urine and faeces with water and flush as soon as possible

Radioactive materials have a reducing 'half life' so that precautions will only need to be carried out for a specific, prescribed period of time. Once the danger of radioactivity is considered negligible, precautions may be discontinued.

It is advisable that staff who have had close contact with radioactive materials should have a shower and a change of clothing when coming off duty, as an extra precaution.

In radiotherapy units, special guidelines may apply and a Geiger counter may be used to assess radioactive levels before disposing of radioactive material.

Relevance to the activities of living

Maintaining a safe environment

The whole concept of isolation nursing is related to maintaining a safe environment for the patient or those who come into contact with him or his fomites.

With infected patients the emphasis is on maintaining a safe environment for other people by preventing spread of the infection. The nursing and medical personnel are the key figures in this.

The safe environment of other hospital staff, e.g. porters and laundry staff, as well as the general public is maintained by safe disposal of infected waste and linen. Bagging and labelling infected blood products for investigation ensures a safe environment for transportation and laboratory staff.

Protective isolation is aimed at maintaining a safe environment for the patient at risk of infection while the treatment for the disease is continued. Once the patient's immune system is able to maintain his own safe environment, isolation procedures can be reduced gradually; initially he may be allowed to eat unsterile food, while staff still wear masks and practise reverse barrier nursing. The patient is then re-introduced to a normal environment over a period of days. During the isolation period it is important that he is not exposed to any known infection. Staff and visitors with colds or sore throats should be excluded at all times, and the reason for this explained.

Radiation isolation is aimed at maintaining a safe environment for those in the vicinity of the radiation, while giving nursing care to the patient.

Appropriate hand washing technique is a most important means of maintaining a safe environment.

Communicating

This activity of living is most influenced by isolation nursing. Isolation immediately affects the normal person-to-person communication process. The patient often becomes depressed and bored because the number of people in contact with him is greatly reduced; visitors are limited and staff limit the number of times they enter and leave the area. The isolation increases when the door to a room is required to be shut and when the door and corridor wall are not made of glass.

The nurses need to be perceptive to the needs of the patient and should discuss with him and his visitors the best way of coping with the isolation problem.

An individual television is a great help, and should be considered essential equipment. A two-way radio or voice link system will enable staff to chat to the patient, and the patient to call the staff, thus reducing the feeling of isolation, but still maintaining the safe environment. A bell must be available so that the patient can summon assistance.

Interests such as reading, crafts, letter writing and jigsaw puzzles should be encouraged as the patient's condition allows. Most articles can be decontaminated, or sterilised as required. Isolation areas should ideally be glass cubicles where the patient can see the outside environment and have a window with an interesting view.

Blood-borne infection such as HIV, has a high media profile. Nurses should be responsible communicators to promote health education on the subject, and should also help to minimise intolerant attitudes by using appropriate verbal and non-verbal communication skills.

Relevance to the
activities of living
continued

Eating and drinking

Some patients are prescribed sterile food and drinks whilst in protective isolation, and these are available in cans, although the patient may find them boring after a while. It is important that the patient maintains an adequate diet while treatment continues. Microwave ovens can sterilise normal food and utensils, so food can be safely prepared in this way. The dietitian should be asked for help as appropriate.

Patients with enteric infections may have an intravenous infusion in situ. When able to eat and drink, individualised or disposable crockery and cutlery should be used.

Eliminating

Ideally all isolation patients should be nursed in a single room with individual toilet and washing facilities. Special precautions are needed for patients who have diarrhoea due to enteric infection.

Personal cleansing and dressing

Patients undergoing source isolation may have to wear hospital garments, or disposable clothes, which may add to the problems of isolation and stigma.

Patients in protective isolation should be encouraged to wear their own freshly laundered day and night clothes. (Arrangements for sterilisation may be necessary.) This will help to encourage individuality and self-esteem.

Controlling body temperature

Patients isolated because of a specific infection should have their temperature recorded 2- or 4-hourly as appropriate, to monitor the course of the infection and associated fever. All necessary equipment for recording should remain within the isolation area. Documentation should remain uncontaminated outside the area.

Expressing sexuality

The whole procedure of isolation may give the patient an impression of having an altered body image, due to the stigma felt by the patient who has an infection. Perceptive and supportive nursing care and good communication skills will help to alleviate the feeling of rejection.

Suggested reading
Ayton M 1984 Protective clothing. What do we use and when? Nursing Times 80(20) May 16: 68–69
Bowell E 1990 Assessing infection risks. Nursing 4(12) June 14: 19–23
Denton F 1986 Psychological and physiological effects of isolation. Nursing 3(3) March: 88–91
Epton V 1990 Salmonella. What risk? Nursing 4(20) October 11: 14–16
Maycock J 1989 An isolating experience: hospital acquired infection. Nursing Times 85(13) March 29: RCN Supplement 75
Room R 1990 The role of the specialist health visitor. Nursing 4(20) October 11: 27–30
Roper N, Logan W, Tierney A 1990 The elements of nursing. 3rd edn. Churchill Livingstone, Edinburgh, pp 67–100
Tierney A (ed) 1986 Clinical nursing practice. Recent advances in nursing 14. Churchill Livingstone, Edinburgh, pp 154–184
Ward K 1988 The role of the infection control nurse. Nursing 3(30) October: 5–8

Communicating

Ear Syringing

Objectives

By the end of this section you should know how to:

- prepare the patient for this procedure
- collect and prepare the equipment
- assist the qualified practitioner to syringe the patient's ear

Related information

Revision of the anatomy and physiology of the external and middle ear.
Review of health authority policy for this procedure.

Some indications for syringing an ear

Syringing an ear is washing out the external auditory canal with a prescribed solution using a special syringe.

This may be required:

- to clear the external canal of an obstruction
- to wash out softened wax

Outline of the procedure

Using the auriscope, the external canal and eardrum are examined. If the eardrum is intact and no other abnormalities are detected, the practice of syringing the ear can be carried out. The syringe is primed with the solution, care being taken to expel all the air. The protective covering is placed over the patient's shoulder and the receiver held in place under the ear. The pinna of the ear is gently pulled in an upwards and backwards direction to straighten out the canal, then the fluid is introduced through the syringe which should point to the roof of the canal so that the solution flows along the roof and down and back out, washing any debris with it (Fig. 2.1). After the qualified practitioner has again examined the canal to assess the result of the syringing, the canal is carefully dried using the dressed applicators.

Figure 2.1
Ear syringing showing fluid being directed to the roof of the aural canal (the nurse should pull the pinna of the ear gently upwards) (Reproduced with permission from Chilman A, Thomas M (eds) 1987 Understanding nursing care, 3rd edn. Churchill Livingstone, Edinburgh)

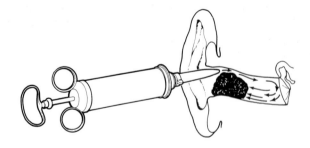

Equipment

Tray
Waterproof protection for the patient
Container with prescribed amount of solution
Aural (ear) syringe
Lotion thermometer
Receiver for return flow
Auriscope
Dressed applicators
Receptacle for soiled disposables

Tap water is commonly used nowadays for ear syringing, although sodium chloride 0.9% or a solution of sodium bicarbonate (4 g to 600 ml water) may be ordered. About 500 ml of the solution is usually prepared.

The temperature of the solution should be 38°C. Temperatures other than this are uncomfortable, may injure tissues and may cause the patient to feel dizzy and nauseated. This procedure is normally only carried out if the tympanic membrane is intact, in which case it is a socially clean procedure.

Guidelines for this nursing practice

- help explain the procedure to the patient and gain his consent and cooperation

- assemble and prepare the equipment

- ensure the patient's privacy

- assist the patient to sit in an upright position with his head tilted slightly to the affected side to aid the return flow of the solution

- observe the patient throughout this activity

- arrange the waterproof protection around the patient's neck and shoulders

- place the receiver for the return flow under his ear and ask for his assistance in holding it in place

- assist the qualified practitioner as requested

- ensure the patient is left feeling as comfortable as possible

- dispose of the equipment safely

- document the procedure appropriately, monitor after-effects and report abnormal findings immediately

Ear Syringing

Relevance to the activities of living

Maintaining a safe environment

Although this does not require aseptic technique, the equipment should be clean or disposable and the nurse should wash her hands before commencing and on completion of the procedure.

It is important to examine the patient's ear before carrying out this procedure as there is a danger of causing serious damage or introducing infection into the middle ear if the tympanic membrane has been ruptured.

The temperature of the solution should be 38°C: cold or hot solutions may stimulate the labyrinth and cause vertigo or nausea.

Communicating

Eardrops (usually oil) may be prescribed for a few days prior to syringing to soften hard cerumen (wax).

It is important to explain to the patient that he may feel slightly dizzy when this procedure is being carried out. If it is being performed to wash away wax which has been impairing the patient's hearing, there should be a marked improvement in hearing afterwards. If the patient wears a hearing aid, the nurse should check that it is working satisfactorily following the practice.

Mobilising

The patient's cooperation in remaining still while the procedure is being carried out is important, as the metal syringe can damage the tissue of the ear.

If there is any evidence of dizziness, the patient may have to rest for a time following the procedure.

Working and playing

Hearing difficulties may prevent the patient carrying out his job efficiently and can also prohibit his participation in or enjoyment of his hobbies and interests.

Suggested reading   Levene B 1983 Hearing loss – the invisible disability. Nursing 2 (18) October: 525–529
Levene B 1985 Sensory loss in the elderly. Nursing 2 (41) September: 1221–1225
Long B, Phipps W 1985 Essentials of medical–surgical nursing – a nursing process approach. C.V. Mosby, St Louis, pp 460–475
Newman D 1990 Assessment of hearing loss in elderly people: the feasibility of a nurse-administered screening test. Journal of Advanced Nursing 15: 400–409
Roper N, Logan W, Tierney A 1990 The elements of nursing, 3rd edn. Churchill Livingstone, Edinburgh, pp 107, 118
Roughneen M 1983 Ear syringing. Nursing 2 (18) October: 530–531
Surkitt-Par D 1989 The removal of foreign bodies. Nursing 3(35) March: 11–14
Verney A 1989 The patient with hearing impairment. Nursing 3(35) March: 17–20

Instillation of Eardrops

Objectives

By the end of this section you should know how to:

- prepare the patient for this nursing practice
- collect and prepare the equipment
- instil drops safely and effectively into the patient's ear

Related information

Revision of the anatomy of the ear.

Revision of administration of medicines, especially checking the medication with the prescription (see p. 12).

Some indications for instilling eardrops

Instillation of eardrops involves dropping a prescribed solution into the external auditory canal from a dropper.

This may be required:

- to soften wax before syringing
- to reduce inflammation and relieve discomfort
- to combat infection

Equipment

Prescribed eardrops
Cotton wool balls
Receptacle for soiled disposables

Guidelines for this nursing practice

- explain the practice to the patient and gain his consent and cooperation
- collect and prepare the equipment
- ensure the patient's privacy
- assist the patient to sit in an upright position with his head tilted slightly away from the affected ear
- observe the patient throughout this activity
- check the drug prescription with the eardrops label
- check the expiry date of the bottle of drops
- verify which ear should receive the drops
- pull the pinna of the ear gently in an upwards and backwards direction in adults, and a downwards and backwards direction in children, to straighten the external canal
- insert the prescribed number of eardrops into the canal
- release the pinna of the ear
- position a piece of cotton wool at the entrance to the canal if this is local policy
- dispose of the equipment safely
- document this nursing practice appropriately, monitor after-effects and report abnormal findings immediately

Relevance to the activities of living

Maintaining a safe environment

To avoid the risk of cross-infection each patient should have an individual container of prescribed eardrops. The nurse should wash her hands before commencing and on completion of the practice.

Communicating

Any patient who is receiving medication by ear may experience difficulty with hearing, and this should be explained.

Should a patient complain of skin irritation, pain or a burning sensation following instillation of an ear medication this should be reported as it may be an indication of a drug allergy.

Mobilising

It aids the effectiveness of the eardrops if the patient avoids tilting his head to the affected side for as long as possible.

Suggested reading

Innes A, Gates N 1985 ENT surgery and disorders. Faber & Faber, London, ch 8
McKenzie G, Chawla H, Gordon D 1986 The special senses, 2nd edn. Churchill Livingstone, Edinburgh, pp 9–47
Surkitt-Par D 1989 The removal of foreign bodies. Nursing 3(35) March: 11–14

Eye Care

There are four parts to this section:

1   **Eye swabbing**
2   **Eye irrigation**
3   **Instillation of eyedrops**
4   **Instillation of eye ointment**

The concluding subsection, 'Relevance to the activities of living', refers to the four practices collectively.

Objectives

By the end of this section you should know how to:

- prepare the patient for these four nursing practices

- collect and prepare the equipment

- carry out eye swabbing, eye irrigation, instillation of eyedrops and instillation of eye ointment

Related information

Revision of the anatomy and physiology of the eye

Revision of administration of medicines (see p. 12) and aseptic technique (see p. 26)

1 EYE SWABBING

Some indications for eye swabbing

- to soothe the eye when a patient is suffering from an insensitive or diseased eye
- to precede the instillation of an eyedrop or the application of an eye ointment
- to remove any eye discharge and/or crusts

Equipment

Sterile eye dressings pack containing a gallipot, small cotton wool balls and a disposable towel

Sterile swabbing solution, e.g. normal saline solution, to soften any crusted discharge

Good light source

Trolley or tray for equipment

Receptacle for soiled disposables

Guidelines for this nursing practice

- explain the practice to the patient and gain his consent and cooperation
- wash the hands
- collect and prepare the equipment
- ensure the patient's privacy
- prepare the patient by helping him into a comfortable position either lying down or seated with his head inclined backwards
- observe the patient throughout this activity
- position the light source to allow maximum observation of the patient's eyes without the beam shining directly into his eyes
- open and arrange the equipment
- wash and dry the hands
- place the disposable towel around the patient's neck
- lightly moisten a cotton wool swab in the prescribed solution
- gently swab from the inner canthus to the outer canthus of the eye using each swab only once. This decreases the risk of cross-infection of one eye to the other or infection of the lacrymal punctum (if both eyes are being swabbed, the healthy eye should be treated first as this again reduces the risk of cross-infection)
- gently dry the patient's eyelids to remove excess moisture
- ensure that the patient is left feeling as comfortable as possible
- dispose of the equipment safely
- document the nursing practice appropriately, monitor after-effects and report any abnormal findings

Eye Care

2 EYE IRRIGATION

Some indications for eye irrigation

Irrigation involves the continuous washing of the eye surface with fluid:

- to aid removal of a corrosive substance from the eye

Equipment

Waterproof sheet
Cotton towel
Sterile eye dressings pack containing a gallipot, small cotton wool balls and a disposable towel
Irrigation fluid, e.g. sterile water, sterile normal saline or universal buffer solution
Lotion thermometer
Irrigating utensil, e.g. undine or intravenous giving set
Receiver for the irrigating fluid
Trolley for equipment
Receptacle for soiled disposables

Guidelines for this nursing practice

- explain the nursing practice to the patient and gain his consent and cooperation

- wash the hands

- collect and prepare the equipment

- ensure the patient's privacy

- observe the patient throughout this activity

- warm the irrigating fluid to 37.8°C

- help the patient into a suitable position either sitting or lying with his head and neck well supported

- apply the waterproof sheet and towel around the patient's neck

- help the patient to turn his head to the side of the affected eye to prevent any (or further) damage of the other eye by the corrosive substance when irrigation is commenced

- wash and dry the hands

- position the receiver below the affected eye against the patient's cheek

- remove any discharge from the eye with a cotton wool ball

- explain to the patient that the flow of fluid is about to begin

- hold the eyelids apart with the first and second fingers

- direct the flow from the irrigator on to the patient's cheek to check that the temperature is comfortable for the patient

- hold the irrigator at a height 2.5 cm above the eye

- direct a steady flow of irrigating fluid from the inner canthus to the outer canthus of the eye

- ask the patient to move his eye up, down and all around to ensure the whole eye is irrigated

- remove the equipment from the patient and ensure that the patient is left feeling as comfortable as possible

- dispose of the equipment safely

- document the nursing practice appropriately, monitor after-effects and report any abnormal findings immediately

3   INSTILLATION OF EYEDROPS

Some indications for instillation of eyedrops

Instillation involves the introduction of a liquid into a cavity drop by drop. In certain disease conditions and following injury eyedrops are prescribed:

- to apply topically a local anaesthetic prior to diagnostic investigations, e.g. tonometry, removal of a foreign body or minor surgery
- to apply topically an antibiotic or anti-inflammatory medicine
- to apply topically a muscle constrictor or dilator to the eye
- to apply topically an artificial lubricant for the eye

Equipment

Sterile eye dressings pack containing a gallipot, small cotton wool balls and a disposable towel

Sterile solution for swabbing

Eyedrops to be administered

Light source

Trolley or tray for equipment

Receptacle for soiled disposables

Eye Care

Guidelines for this nursing practice

- explain the nursing practice to the patient and gain his consent and cooperation
- wash the hands
- collect and prepare the equipment
- ensure the patient's privacy
- observe the patient throughout this activity
- help the patient into a comfortable position
- position the light source
- check the medicine prescription with the eyedrops label
- check the expiry date of the bottle of drops
- verify which eye should receive the drops
- wash and dry the hands
- swab the eye clean if a discharge is present
- hold a swab in the non-dominant hand under the lower lid margin to remove excess moisture after the drop instillation
- ask the patient to look up and evert the lower lid
- hold the dropper in the dominant hand, about 2 cm above the eye, and allow one drop to fall into the lower conjunctival sac (Fig. 2.2)
- ask the patient to close his eye then remove excess moisture
- ensure that the patient is left feeling as comfortable as possible
- dispose of the equipment safely
- document the nursing practice appropriately, monitor after-effects and report any abnormal findings immediately

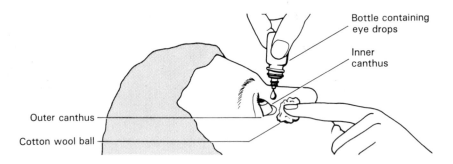

Figure 2.2
Instillation of eyedrops: the lower lid is pulled gently downwards to create a pouch into which the drop is placed

Bottle containing eye drops

Inner canthus

Outer canthus

Cotton wool ball

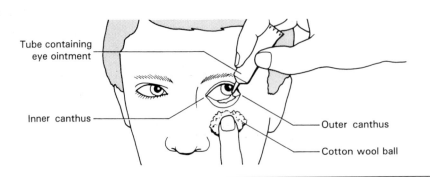

Figure 2.3
Instillation of eye ointment: the lower lid is pulled gently downwards to create a pouch into which the ointment is placed

Tube containing eye ointment

Inner canthus

Outer canthus

Cotton wool ball

4   INSTILLATION OF EYE OINTMENT

Some indications for instillation of eye ointment

In certain disease conditions, and following injury, eye ointment is prescribed:

- to instil a medicine topically in place of eyedrops when a prolonged action of the medicine is required

- to form a protective film over the corneal surface of an eye

- to act as a soothing agent for the patient suffering from an inflamed eye or lid margin

Equipment

Sterile eye dressings pack containing a gallipot, small cotton wool balls and a disposable towel
Sterile solution for swabbing
Eye ointment to be administered
Trolley or tray for equipment
Light source
Receptacle for soiled disposables

Guidelines for this nursing practice

- explain the nursing practice to the patient and gain his consent and cooperation

- wash the hands

- collect and prepare the equipment

- ensure the patient's privacy

- observe the patient throughout this activity

- help the patient into a comfortable position

- position the light source

- check the medicine prescription with the eye ointment label

- check the expiry date of the tube of ointment

- verify which eye should receive the ointment

- wash and dry the hands

- swab the eye clean to remove all traces of the previously instilled ointment and/or discharge

- hold a swab in the non-dominant hand under the lower lid margin to remove excess ointment after instillation

- ask the patient to look up and evert the lower lid

- hold the tube of ointment in the dominant hand

- with the nozzle of the tube 2.5 cm above the lower lid, squeeze the tube to allow a ribbon of ointment to run into the lower conjunctival sac from the inner canthus to the outer canthus (Fig. 2.3)

- ask the patient to close his eye then remove excess ointment

- inform the patient that he may experience blurred vision for a few minutes following the instillation of the ointment

- ensure that the patient is left feeling as comfortable as possible

- dispose of the equipment safely

- document the nursing practice appropriately, monitor after-effects and report any abnormal findings immediately

Eye Care

Relevance to the
activities of living

Maintaining a safe environment

To reduce the potential risk of cross-infection when caring for a patient's eye, the nurse must wash her hands thoroughly and swab the cleaner eye first from the inner canthus to the outer canthus. Use sterile swabbing solutions where possible, but in the case of an emergency, tap water may be used. Multiple-dose containers of eye medication should be changed regularly, to reduce the risk of cross-infection; usually, each patient has eyedrops or a tube of ointment reserved for his use alone.

When an eyedrop or ointment is to be instilled, care must be taken not to touch the eye surface with the applicator as this could cause injury to the eye and contamination of the applicator. If an eyedrop and eye ointment are to be instilled at the same time, the eyedrop should be instilled first. The greasy/oily base of an ointment once applied would prevent the absorption of the medicine within the eyedrop. The nurse is responsible for instilling the correct medicine into the correct eye. Any discrepancy must be reported immediately.

If the patient's vision is impaired, the nurse should assist the patient in maintaining a safe environment during his stay in hospital, and help to identify problems which may occur following discharge.

Should a patient need to continue eye medication following discharge, the nurse will assess and teach him or a relative to become competent in the practice. Self-administration of eyedrops can be assisted with the use of a clip-on plastic device known as Autodrop.

Communicating

The nurse should explain the procedure simply to the patient and inform him of her intended actions. When an emergency eye irrigation is to be performed the nurse must be quick and precise with the explanation, so that the time the corrosive substance is in the patient's eye is minimised. When a patient is extremely anxious or in severe pain the medical practitioner may prescribe local anaesthetic drops.

Should a patient complain of skin irritation, pain or a burning sensation following instillation of an eye medication this should be reported as it may indicate a drug allergy. Following the instillation of an eye ointment the nurse must warn the patient that his vision will be blurred for 5–6 minutes due to the greasy/oily base of the ointment.

Due to the injury, disease or the effect of the topical medicine, the patient's previous range of vision may be impaired temporarily or permanently. The nurse will need to assist the patient to adapt to this change.

When a patient wears spectacles the nurse should assist the patient in the application and care of the spectacles according to his wishes.

Expressing sexuality

Due to the visual appearance of some eye diseases or the effect of trauma to the eye, a patient may develop a negative body image, with resultant effects on his selfesteem. He should be helped to come to terms with this altered body image, whether short-lived or permanent.

If vision in both eyes is suddenly impaired for any reason, many other ALs will be affected and the patient will require help to adapt to this sudden loss of independence.

Suggested reading

Bocking H, Sercombe A, Kenny M et al 1990 Making sense of artificial eyes. Nursing Times 86(18) May 2: 40–41

Brooks J 1989 The red eye – 1. Practice Nurse 2(2) June: 73–75

Brooks J 1989 The red eye – 2. Practice Nurse 2(5) October: 226–230

Brunner L, Suddarth D 1988 Textbook of medical–surgical nursing, 6th edn. Lippincott, Philadelphia, pp 1343–1347

Hughes-Lamb B 1981 Caring for the visually handicapped. Nursing 1(28) August: 1221–1224

Josse E 1984 Corneal abscess from soft contact lenses. Nursing Times Journal of Infection Control Nursing 80(37) September 12: 3–4

Lloyd F 1990 Making sense of eye care. Nursing Times 86(1) January 3: 36–37

Roper N, Logan W, Tierney A 1990 The elements of nursing, 3rd edn. Churchill Livingstone, Edinburgh, pp 105–106, 119

Smith J 1983 Ophthalmic problems in general nursing. Nursing 2(17) September: 507–508

Smith S 1987 Drugs and the eye. Nursing Times 83(25) June 24: 48–50

Removal of Nasal Packing

Objectives

By the end of this section you should know how to:

- prepare the patient for this nursing practice
- collect and prepare the equipment
- describe the method used to remove nasal packing

Related information

Revision of the anatomy of the nose.

Review of health authority policy for this nursing practice.

Some indications for nasal packing

Nasal packing is inserted by a medical practitioner and usually consists of long strips of ribbon gauze, which may be impregnated with medication, being introduced and packed tightly into the nasal cavities (Fig. 2.4).

This may be required:

- to help prevent haemorrhage or haematoma after some surgical procedures to the nose
- to treat some cases of epistaxis. Epistat catheters are increasingly the equipment of choice to treat epistaxis (Fig. 2.5)

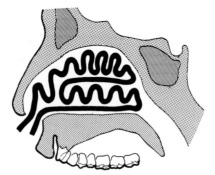

Figure 2.4
Position of nasal packing (Reproduced with permission from Chilman A, Thomas M (eds) 1987 Understanding nursing care, 3rd edn. Churchill Livingstone, Edinburgh)

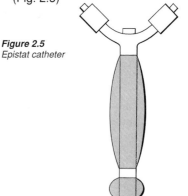

Figure 2.5
Epistat catheter

Equipment

Trolley or tray
Sterile metal dissecting forceps
Bowl to receive removed packing
Protective covering for the patient
Sterile Q-tips
Sterile gallipot
Sachet of normal saline
Icepack
Receptacle for soiled disposables

Guidelines for this nursing practice

- explain the nursing practice to the patient and gain his consent and cooperation
- collect and prepare the equipment
- ensure the patient's privacy
- assist the patient to sit as comfortably as possible in an upright position in bed
- observe the patient throughout this activity
- place the protective covering around the patient's chest
- ask the patient to hold the bowl at chin level to receive the removed packing
- hold the end of the packing with the dissecting forceps and exert a gentle pull to start removing the pack. Metal dissecting forceps are preferable for this procedure as they are stronger than the disposable plastic variety. If the nose has been tightly packed it is sometimes necessary to use quite a bit of pressure to remove the packing
- pause, if requested by the patient
- observe for signs of bleeding after the packing has been removed
- deflate the balloons on the catheter in the same way as the balloon in a self-retaining urinary catheter

- observe the patient for evidence of epistaxis
- after at least 30 minutes, if there is no evidence, gently withdraw the catheter
- explain to the patient the necessity for staying in bed for the next 2 hours, refraining from bending his head unnecessarily, and from blowing his nose for the next 24 hours. Some schools of thought suggest placing an icepack over the patient's nose during the 2 hours bedrest; others consider this unnecessary unless there is evidence of bleeding. Gentle cleaning with normal saline and Q-tips immediately after removing the packing is the policy in some areas but in others this is not recommended for the first couple of hours, as it is thought the action may induce bleeding
- ensure that the patient is left feeling as comfortable as possible
- dispose of the equipment safely
- document this nursing practice appropriately, monitor after-effects and report abnormal findings immediately

Removal of Nasal Packing

Relevance to the activities of living

Maintaining a safe environment

To help prevent cross-infection the nurse should wash her hands before commencing and on completion of this nursing practice.

Communicating

The presence of nasal packing can cause a problem with verbal communication because the passage of air is impeded and the patient's normal ability to control sound is impaired.

The patient may feel faint when the pack is being removed and if the pack is large some discomfort and pain may be experienced. An analgesic or sedative may be administered prior to its removal.

Epistat catheters can be more effective than packing in applying pressure to bleeding points. They cause less discomfort when being removed.

Breathing

While the packing is in his nose the patient is forced to mouth breathe and after the packing has been removed it can take some time for him to return to breathing through his nose, so this delayed action should be discussed with the patient.

Eating and drinking

While the nasal packing is in place and mouth breathing necessary, eating and drinking can present some problems, because swallowing has to be more consciously controlled.

Personal cleansing and dressing

Because the patient is forced to mouth breathe, frequent appropriate mouthcare should be offered while nasal packing is in situ.

Mobilising

After the removal of the nasal pack, the possibility of bleeding recurring should be explained to the patient; resting for 24 hours helps to reduce the possibility of further haemorrhage.

Suggested reading   Innes A, Gates N 1985 ENT surgery and disorders. Faber & Faber, London, ch 13
Roper N, Logan W, Tierney A 1990 The elements of nursing, 3rd edn. Churchill
      Livingstone, Edinburgh, pp 136–138
Sealey L 1985 Nasal obstruction. Nursing Mirror 161(5) July 31: 22–24

Neurological Examination

Objectives

By the end of this section you should know how to:

- prepare the patient for a neurological examination
- collect and prepare the equipment
- assist the medical practitioner during neurological examination if required

Related information

Revision of the anatomy and physiology of the nervous system.

Revision of care of the unconscious patient (see p. 312).

Some indications for neurological examination

Neurological examination is a method of obtaining some objective data in relation to the function of a patient's nervous system. This may be required:

- to aid in the diagnosis of a neurological disease
- to monitor the effect of a neurological disease
- to aid in the assessment of treatment during the course of a neurological disease

Outline of the procedure

This procedure is carried out by a medical practitioner usually in conjunction with an examination of the motor and sensory function of the patient's trunk and limbs. The ophthalmoscope and pencil torch are used to assess the function of the optic, the oculomotor, the trochlear and the ophthalmic branch of the trigeminal cranial nerves. The auriscope and tuning fork are used to examine the ears and assess the function of the vestibulocochlear cranial nerve, respectively. Assessment of the patient's sensation to pain, touch and temperature are estimated by using a sterile needle, a cotton wool ball and the test tubes of hot and cold water. The olfactory cranial nerve is assessed when the patient is asked to identify the odours of the various strong-smelling substances. The tendon hammer is used by the medical practitioner when testing a spinal reflex such as the knee jerk. Assessment for an upper motor neurone lesion will also require the use of a tendon hammer for the act of stroking the lateral aspect of the sole of the patient's foot. The function of the facial cranial nerve is assessed by asking the patient to identify various substances, i.e. salt, sugar, vinegar and lemon juice. The patient will be required to use the mouth rinse after each substance is tasted to prevent inaccurate results.

Equipment

Ophthalmoscope
Pencil torch
Auriscope
Tuning fork
Sterile injection needle
Non-sterile cotton wool balls
Test tubes filled with hot and cold water
Small containers of various strong-smelling substances, e.g. peppermint, oil of cloves
Tendon hammer
Small samples of salt, sugar, lemon juice and vinegar

Glass of water for rinsing the patient's mouth
Trolley or tray for equipment
Receptacle for used mouth rinse
Receptacle for soiled disposables

Guidelines for this nursing practice

- help to explain the procedure to the patient and gain his consent and cooperation
- wash the hands
- prepare the equipment
- ensure the patient's privacy
- observe the patient throughout this activity
- help the patient into a comfortable position

- assist the medical practitioner during the examination if required
- ensure the patient is left feeling as comfortable as possible
- dispose of the equipment safely
- document the procedure appropriately, monitor after-effects and report abnormal findings immediately

Relevance to the activities of living

Maintaining a safe environment

All equipment should be clean or disposable and all precautions taken to prevent cross-infection. The nurse should wash her hands before commencing and on completion of the nursing practice.

A nurse is not always present during a neurological examination, but assistance may be required by the medical practitioner, for example with a paralysed or unconscious patient.

Communicating

The medical practitioner who carries out the examination gives the patient an explanation of the procedure, but the nurse may be required to repeat the explanation.

Depending on the nature of the disease condition which requires the neurological examination (and they are many and diverse), any of the patient's activities of living may be affected, but the examination itself does not have any adverse effects on ALs.

Suggested reading

Brunner L, Suddarth D 1988 Textbook of medical–surgical nursing. 6th edn. Lippincott, Philadelphia pp 1401–1406
Darwin J 1980 Assessing levels of consciousness. Nursing 1 (15) July: 672–673
Long B, Phipps W 1985 Essentials of medical–surgical nursing – a nursing process approach. C.V. Mosby, St Louis, p 359
Roper N, Logan W, Tierney A 1990 The elements of nursing, 3rd edn. Churchill Livingstone, Edinburgh, ch 7

Lumbar Puncture

Objectives

By the end of this section you should know how to:

- prepare the patient for this nursing practice
- collect and prepare the equipment
- assist the medical practitioner to perform a lumbar puncture

Related information

Revision of the anatomy and physiology of the brain and spinal cord, with special reference to the cerebrospinal fluid and the meninges.

Revision of the anatomy of the lumbar vertebrae.

Revision of aseptic technique (see p. 26).

Some indications for lumbar puncture

Lumbar puncture is the insertion of a specialised needle into the lumbar subarachnoid space to gain access to the cerebrospinal fluid (CSF).

This may be required:

- to obtain a sample of cerebrospinal fluid for investigative and diagnostic purposes, e.g.:
  — bacteriological investigation for patients suspected of having meningitis or encephalitis
  — cytological investigation for patients suspected of having a malignant tumour
  — to identify the presence of blood in the cerebrospinal fluid following trauma or a suspected subarachnoid haemorrhage
- to introduce radio-opaque fluid into the subarachnoid space for radiographic investigation
- to identify raised intraspinal/intracranial pressure and provide relief if appropriate by removing some of the cerebrospinal fluid
- to introduce intrathecal medication such as cytotoxic agents or antibiotics

Outline of the procedure

A lumbar puncture is performed by a medical practitioner using aseptic technique. The patient is helped into the correct position. An area of skin above the 3rd, 4th and 5th lumbar vertebrae is prepared and cleaned with antiseptic solution prior to the administration of local anaesthesia. A special lumbar puncture needle is inserted between the 3rd and 4th lumbar vertebrae or 4th and 5th lumbar vertebrae in order to gain access to the subarachnoid space below the spinal cord in the region of the cauda equina (Fig. 2.6). Once in position the stilette of the needle is removed. A manometer is attached to the end of the needle via a two-way tap and the cerebrospinal fluid is allowed to flow into the manometer to record intraspinal pressure. At this stage the medical practitioner may require Queckenstedt's test to be performed (see p. 69).

When pressure recordings are completed the manometer is occluded, and 2 or 3 ml of cerebrospinal fluid is allowed to flow into three separate sterile specimen containers as required while still maintaining asepsis. The medical practitioner will note the colour, consistency and opacity of the cerebrospinal fluid as well as observing the presence or absence of blood. On completion the needle is removed and the puncture site is covered by a small sterile dressing or plastic sealant spray. The patient remains lying flat in bed for 6–12 hours following this procedure and appropriate observations are maintained during this period.

The position of the patient

The correct position is important for the success and safety of this procedure. The patient should lie on his side on a firm bed with one pillow. He should stretch his lumbar vertebrae by flexing his head and neck and drawing his knees up to his abdomen, holding them with his hands (Fig. 2.7). The nurse can assist by supporting the patient behind the knees and the neck, and helping to maintain the extension of the lumbar vertebrae, thus widening the intervertebral space. This will help to ensure that the insertion and correct placement of the lumbar puncture needle is safely achieved. Once the needle is in position the medical practitioner may ask the patient to slowly straighten his legs without moving the position of his back. This will reduce the intraabdominal pressure which can cause an abnormal reading of intraspinal pressure.

Very occasionally this procedure is performed with a patient sitting straddled on a chair and facing the back of the chair with his head resting on folded arms. This position may be chosen by the medical practitioner when performing a lumbar puncture on a very obese patient or a dyspnoeic patient.

Figure 2.6
Lumbar puncture: position of the needle in relation to the vertebrae

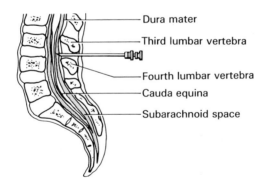

- Dura mater
- Third lumbar vertebra
- Fourth lumbar vertebra
- Cauda equina
- Subarachnoid space

Figure 2.7
Lumbar puncture: position of the patient

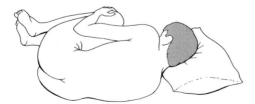

Lumbar Puncture

Equipment

Trolley

Sterile dressings pack

Sterile drapes

Sterile surgical gloves for the medical practitioner

Sterile lumbar puncture set containing:

— lumbar puncture needle

— spinal manometer

— two-way tap

Alcohol-based antiseptic lotion for cleansing the skin

Local anaesthetic and equipment for its administration

Syringe and needles for local anaesthetic

Sterile dressing, e.g. Airstrip or plastic sealant spray

Three sterile specimen containers appropriately labelled, completed laboratory forms, and plastic specimen bag for transportation. These may be required for three separate samples of CSF for microbiological, biochemical and cytological investigation.

Watch with seconds hand for Queckenstedt's test

Receptacle for disposables

Lumbar puncture needle

This is a rigid stainless steel needle 5 cm (approx) in length, complete with its own sharp pointed stilette; this helps the entry of the needle into the correct position. Once the stilette is removed, the blunt end of the needle lies within the subarachnoid space, and should cause no damage to tissue during the procedure. Needles are usually supplied with their own metal two-way tap, but a Luer disposable tap may be used.

Guidelines for this nursing practice

- help to explain the procedure to the patient and gain his consent and cooperation
- ensure the patient's privacy
- help to collect and prepare the equipment
- help to prepare the sterile field
- help the patient into the appropriate position, and remain with him to maintain that position
- observe the patient throughout this activity
- help to expose the lumbar region of the patient's back, and assist the medical practitioner as required
- encourage the patient to breathe quietly in order to prevent any hyperventilation which gives a false low pressure reading
- assist the medical practitioner with the Queckenstedt's test if required by compressing the jugular vein, or veins, as directed

- hold the appropriate sterile containers to receive the flow of CSF as directed, maintaining asepsis
- ensure that the puncture site is covered with a sterile dressing or plastic sealant spray once the needle is removed
- help the patient into a comfortable position lying flat with only one pillow, once the procedure is completed, explaining the importance of maintaining this position for 6–12 hours following the procedure
- ensure the patient is left feeling as comfortable as possible with everything he requires at hand
- dispose of the equipment safely
- document the procedure appropriately, monitor after-effects, and report abnormal findings immediately
- dispatch the labelled CSF specimens to the laboratory with their completed forms immediately

Queckenstedt's test

This test is performed to determine whether or not there is an obstruction in the spinal subarachnoid pathway. This may be due to a fractured or dislocated vertebra, or a tumour. Normally there is a rapid rise in intraspinal pressure when jugular compression is applied and an equally rapid return to normal when pressure is released. Any obstruction will cause a much slower rise and fall of the intraspinal pressure. The test is only performed to investigate a spinal lesion. It is never performed when any intracranial lesion is suspected, as raised intracranial pressure could increase the risk of brain damage.

The medical practitioner will ask for jugular compression to be applied for the maximum of 10 seconds and released for 10 seconds. Pressure readings are recorded for each 10 second interval.

Lumbar Puncture

Relevance to the activities of living

Maintaining a safe environment

This is an invasive procedure which involves direct access to the spinal and brain tissue via the cerebrospinal fluid. Asepsis should be maintained during and following the procedure and adequate hand washing technique should be practised to prevent cross-infection. The puncture site should be observed for any evidence of localised infection or leakage, and accurate observations of the patient's condition will help to monitor any evidence of developing infection.

A lumbar puncture is performed as a neurological investigation. A patient who is confused or disorientated may need cot sides on the bed to prevent falls and maintain the safety of his environment.

A lumbar puncture should not be performed if raised intracranial pressure is suspected. The raised pressure may cause the brainstem tissue to herniate through the foramen magnum. This is known as 'coning' and could be fatal.

Safety of staff transporting specimens should be maintained by enclosing containers in plastic specimen bags (see Specimen collection, p. 198).

Communicating

The patient should lie horizontally with only one pillow, either supine or on his side. This will minimise the effect of changes in intraspinal pressure caused by the removal of 1–3 ml of CSF during the procedure, and help to prevent any headache or dizziness occurring. This position is usually maintained for 6–12 hours, depending on the patient's condition. There is, however, conflicting evidence about the length of time the patient needs to remain horizontal following this procedure.

The patient's general condition should be noted, e.g. orientation, restlessness, drowsiness, nausea.

Any evidence of cerebral irritability should be observed. Fitting, twitching, spasticity or weakness of limb movements should be reported immediately and recorded.

The patient's level of consciousness should be recorded as prescribed, depending on his condition. Neurological observations should be maintained for 18–24 hours following this investigation. (see care of the unconscious patient p. 312).

The patient may complain of a headache following this procedure. Analgesic medication should be administered as prescribed. The nurse should be observant for any non-verbal communication indicating pain, and anticipate the patient's needs as appropriate. The fact that the patient might experience discomfort should be explained to him.

Breathing

The pulse, respiration and blood pressure should be recorded 4-hourly, or as indicated by the patient's condition. Abnormalities may indicate developing infection, or evidence of cerebral changes, and should be reported immediately.

Eating and drinking

A normal diet may be ordered as the patient's condition allows. However, while he is lying flat some adjustments and help may be needed. An adequate fluid intake should be maintained following the procedure. Drinks should be easily accessible to the patient, and specialised cups or straws used as appropriate.

Eliminating

It may be necessary for the patient to use a urinal/bedpan instead of a commode for a period following the procedure because of the 6–12 hours bedrest, and the reason for this should be explained to the patient.

Controlling body temperature

The temperature should be monitored for as long as necessary following the procedure. Four-hourly recordings should be maintained for 48 hours and any rise in temperature which might indicate a developing infection should be reported.

Mobilising

The patient should remain flat in bed for 6–12 hours following the procedure to prevent headache or dizziness. Mobilising should initially commence with the patient sitting up in bed for a period of time before progressing to further activity, as his condition allows. This will reduce any further risk of headaches or dizziness which can occur if the patient changes his position too rapidly following this procedure.

Suggested reading

Allan D 1989 Making sense of ... Lumbar puncture. Nursing Times 85(49) December 6: 39–42

Allan D (ed) 1988 Nursing and the neurosciences. Churchill Livingstone, Edinburgh, pp 54–56

Bass B, Vandervoort M K 1988 Post lumbar puncture headache. Canadian Nurse 84(4): 15–18

Carpaat P, Vancrevel H 1981 Lumbar puncture headache. Controlled study. The Lancet 8256(11) November 21: 1133–1134

Roper N, Logan W, Tierney A 1990 The elements of nursing, 3rd edn. Churchill Livingstone, Edinburgh, pp 116–128

Quigley J et al 1989 Neurological investigations. Nursing 3(33) January: 12–17

Section 3

Breathing

Respiration

Objectives

By the end of this section you should know how to:

- assess, measure and record respirations

Related information

Revision of the anatomy and physiology of the respiratory system.

Some indications for assessing respiration

Respiration is the exchange of oxygen and carbon dioxide between the cells of the body and the environment through rhythmic expansion and deflation of the lungs. A respiration consists of an inhalation, an exhalation and the pause which follows.

The respiration rate may be assessed for the following reasons:

- on admission: to ascertain if the respiration rate, depth and pattern is within normal range for the patient's age

- preoperatively: to ascertain the patient's baseline respiration rate, depth and pattern

- postoperatively: to monitor the rate, depth and pattern and compare the findings with the baseline data

- to monitor the patient's condition during and after, for example:
  — aspiration of the pleural cavity
  — pleural biopsy
  — peritoneal dialysis

- to estimate the degree of dysfunction on admission and the effect of treatment on, for example:
  — patients who have cardiopulmonary disease
  — patients who have a head injury

Equipment

Watch with a seconds hand

Guidelines for this nursing practice

- ensure that the patient is as relaxed and comfortable as possible and unaware of the counting process

- count the respiratory rate and observe the depth and pattern immediately after counting the pulse rate and while still holding the patient's wrist

- count the number of respirations for at least 30 seconds. If any abnormality is suspected, respirations should be assessed for a full minute

- document the results appropriately, comparing past recordings, and report abnormal findings immediately

Relevance to the activities of living

Communicating

Patients with respiratory abnormalities may have difficulty with verbal communication. A bell to enable the patient to summon assistance is essential and a writing pad and pencil may be helpful.

Breathing

The rate, depth and pattern of respiration should be observed.

Rate: Normal respiratory rates vary according to age. The accepted normal range for the various age groups is:

healthy adults	14–20 per minute
adolescents	18–22 per minute
children	22–28 per minute
infants	30 or more per minute

The relationship of pulse and respiration is fairly constant in healthy people. The ratio is one respiration to every four or five heart beats.

Depth: The depth of respiration is approximately the same for each person, although the amount of air exchanged can vary enormously. The depth of respiration is described as normal, shallow or deep.

Pattern: A normal breathing pattern is effortless, evenly paced, regular and automatic. Some abnormal patterns are described as:

- *dyspnoea*, which is difficult and laboured breathing: dilated nostrils are often apparent and the entire chest wall and shoulder girdle are raised and lowered in an exaggerated manner
- *Cheyne–Stokes* respirations, which involve a gradual increase in the depth of respiration followed by a gradual decrease, then a period of no breathing, known as apnoea; this syndrome may be associated with terminal illness
- *Kussmaul's* respirations, which involve an increased rate and depth with panting and long grunting expirations; this syndrome may be associated with lobar pneumonia
- *stertorous* respirations, which refer to noisy respirations, usually caused by excessive secretions in the trachea or bronchi
- *stridor*, which is the name given to the harsh, high-pitched sound on inspiration usually caused by laryngeal obstruction

There is some voluntary control of the rate and depth of respirations. Patients with a respiratory dysfunction may be taught breathing exercises to control respiration and permit the optimum benefit of oxygen intake within the limitations of the dysfunction.

Eating and drinking

Respiratory abnormalities can cause difficulty in eating and drinking, because it is not possible to swallow and breathe at the same time. Soft, moist food should be offered and the patient should be encouraged to drink fluids through a straw as this helps him to synchronise more easily his breathing and swallowing.

Relevance to the
activities of living
continued

Eliminating

Patients who are breathless may need assistance in using a bedpan or in getting to the commode or toilet. The difficulty they experience in mobilising and the related anxiety of urinal or faecal soiling can exacerbate the breathlessness. On the other hand, the associated anxiety may be conducive to constipation, and the eventual straining at stool may also aggravate the breathless state.

Personal cleansing and dressing

Patients who have breathing problems may need assistance with washing and dressing. Light, loose clothing should be worn so that chest and abdominal movement is not restricted.

Controlling body temperature

One of the results of pyrexia is an increase in respiration rate as the body attempts to rid itself of excess heat. Hypothermia results in slowing of the respiratory rate.

Mobilising

Exertion results in an increased respiratory rate and when there is already dysfunction, may cause distress. Correct positioning of the patient in bed or in a chair can help alleviate some of the respiratory distress. The reduction in mobility may be conducive to constipation, which in turn may aggravate an already breathless state.

Working and playing

Patients who have breathing problems may be unable to continue in their current employment and with their present hobbies and interests.

Sleeping

The upright position which is preferred by patients with severe breathlessness may not be conducive to sleep, and the physiological changes associated with the disease may have an adverse effect on the sleep centre in the hypothalamus.

Dying

Cheyne–Stokes respirations often occur with the approach of death, when the body mechanisms, including respiratory control, become increasingly impaired.

Suggested reading   Boylan A, Brown P 1985 Respirations: observations. Nursing Times 81(11) March
13: 35–38
Glover A 1986 Hyperventilation. Nursing Times 82(49) December 3: 54–55
Hamilton H (ed) 1985 Nurse's reference library – procedures. Springhouse
Corporation, Pennsylvania, pp 14–16
Hanning C 1986 Sleep and breathing – to sleep, perchance to breathe. Intensive Care
Nursing 2(1): 8–15
Knepil J 1983 The control of breathing. Nursing Mirror 156 (19) May 11: 44–46
Roper N, Logan W, Tierney A 1990 The elements of nursing, 3rd edn. Churchill
Livingstone, Edinburgh, pp 145–148

Pulse

Objectives

By the end of this section you should know how to:

- prepare the patient for this nursing practice
- locate, assess, measure and record the radial pulse
- locate the major pulse points of the body

Related information

Revision of the anatomy and physiology of the cardiovascular system, particularly the heart and main arteries.

Some indications for assessing the radial pulse

A pulse is the rhythmic expansion and recoil of the elastic arteries caused by the ejection of blood from the left ventricle. It can be palpated where an artery near the body surface can be pressed against a firm structure, e.g. bone. It may be assessed for the following reasons:

- arranged admission: to ascertain the patient's pulse and assess whether or not it is within the normal range for the person's age
- emergency admission: to ascertain if the pulse is within the normal range for the person's age
- to correlate pulse data with temperature readings when the temperature is elevated
- to help estimate, in general terms, the degree of fluid loss when the level of body fluids is lowered, e.g. after excessive vomiting, excessive diarrhoea, haemorrhage
- preoperatively: to ascertain the patient's baseline pulse rate, rhythm and quality
- postoperatively: to monitor the rate, rhythm and quality as indicators of the patient's condition and to compare the findings with the baseline data
- to estimate the degree of dysfunction on admission, and the effect of treatment on:
  — patients who have cardiovascular disease
  — patients who have pulmonary disease

Equipment

Watch with a seconds hand

Guidelines for this nursing practice

- explain the nursing practice to the patient and obtain his consent and cooperation

- ensure that the patient is in a position which is as comfortable and relaxed as possible

- observe the patient throughout this activity

- locate the radial artery, place the first and second fingers along it and press gently

- count the pulse for 60 seconds to allow sufficient time to detect any irregularities or other defects

- document the findings appropriately, comparing past recordings, and report abnormal findings immediately

Sites of major pulse points of the body

Although the pulse assessment is usually made using the radial artery, there are other sites where an artery near the body surface can be pressed against an underlying bone, or other firm body structure. The other major sites are (Fig. 3.1):
— temporal
— carotid
— brachial
— radial
— femoral
— popliteal
— posterior tibial
— dorsalis pedis

Figure 3.1
Major pulse points

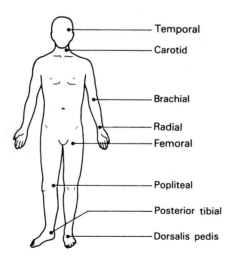

Temporal
Carotid
Brachial
Radial
Femoral
Popliteal
Posterior tibial
Dorsalis pedis

Pulse

Relevance to the activities of living

Breathing

Rate: The resting adult will normally have a pulse rate of between 60–100 beats per minute. Tachycardia (rapid pulse rate) can be a result of pain, anger, fear or anxiety, all of which stimulate the sympathetic nervous system. It can also occur in some heart diseases, anaemia, fever and during exercise, all of which require greater amounts of oxygen and so increase the cardiac output. Bradycardia (slow pulse rate) occurs in any condition which stimulates the parasympathetic nervous system; it also occurs in fit athletes, who develop a very efficient heart muscle action.

Rhythm: The rhythm should be regular and any irregularities should be noted. It should be observed whether the irregularities occur at regular or irregular intervals.

Quality: The pulse pressure is the difference between systolic and diastolic pressure. The force is a reflection of the pulse strength. The pulse is usually recorded as being normal, bounding, weak and thready, or absent.

Elasticity: The elastic recoil of the artery wall should be noted. The artery of a healthy young adult feels flexible and non-tortuous; quite different from that of an elderly patient suffering from, e.g. arteriosclerosis, whose artery will feel hard and cord-like.

The pulse rate is much higher in babies and young children than in adults, because they have a higher metabolic rate. In children and young adults it is fairly common to find an irregular increase in rate on inspiration and decrease on expiration. Occasionally a pacemaker 'fires' before the sinoatrial node and the resulting decrease in filling time of the heart chambers causes a pause in the rhythm which can be detected when assessing the pulse.

Eating and drinking

The level of the body fluids can affect the pulse rate as can electrolyte imbalance.

A drop in the level of body fluids, e.g. as a result of haemorrhage, will lead to a rapid, thready and weak pulse. Severe electrolyte imbalance will cause impaired cell function and will cause cardiac arrhythmias.

Controlling body temperature

As mentioned previously, fever causes the rate of the pulse to be raised because of the need for greater supplies of oxygen. Hypothermia can cause a slowing down of the rate because of the need to keep the body's core temperature as high as possible.

Mobilising

Exercise increases the rate of the pulse, because of the increased demand from muscles for oxygen and nutrients, and the increased production of waste products.

Working and playing

Occupations which demand physical exertion will result in an increased pulse rate, as will hobbies such as active participation in sport.

Dying

The peripheral pulses are often difficult to palpate in the dying patient because of the gradual non-function of the various cardiopulmonary mechanisms, and may be absent in the period immediately prior to death.

Suggested reading
Hamilton H (ed) 1985 Nurse's reference library – procedures. Springhouse Corporation, Pennsylvania, pp 14–16

Nursing Standard 1988 Finger on the pulse. Nursing Standard (Wall Chart) 2(47) August 27: 22–23

Roper N, Logan W, Tierney A 1990 The elements of nursing, 3rd edn. Churchill Livingstone, Edinburgh, pp 139–140

Apical–radial Pulses

Objectives

By the end of this section you should know how to:

- prepare the patient for this nursing practice
- locate, assess, measure and record the apical–radial pulses

Related information

Revision of the anatomy and physiology of the cardiovascular system.

Revision of pulse (see p. 78).

Some indications for assessing the apical–radial pulses

The rate at the apex of the heart and the radial pulse rate are counted simultaneously and compared to ascertain if there is a deficit in the rate. It may be assessed for the following reasons:

- to estimate the degree of dysfunction on admission and the effect of treatment on:
  — patients who have cardiac impairment
  — patients who are receiving medication to improve heart action
  — patients who have vascular disease

Equipment

Watch with a seconds hand
Stethoscope

Guidelines for this nursing practice

Two nurses are required to carry out this practice.

- explain the nursing practice to the patient and gain his consent and cooperation
- ensure the patient's privacy
- collect the equipment
- assist the patient to a comfortable position so that there is easy access to his chest wall
- observe the patient throughout this activity
- place the diaphragm of the stethoscope over the apex of the heart (Fig. 3.2). This is usually located at the 5th intercostal space and 12 cm left of the midline (nurse 1)

- locate the radial pulse (nurse 2)
- ensure that the watch is visible to both nurses who begin counting the rates simultaneously for 1 minute
- document the results appropriately, compare past recordings, and report abnormal findings immediately

Relevance to the activities of living

Breathing

The patient who has a radial pulse deficit because of heart disease may have an elevated respiratory rate, because the inefficient heart action eventually leads to pulmonary oedema which causes respiratory distress.

The rate at the apex and at the radial artery should be compared. If there is a deficit in the radial pulse it should be reported as it may indicate left ventricular failure.

Controlling body temperature

An impaired blood supply to the limbs will probably result in complaints of cold hands and feet. The wearing of gloves and socks should be encouraged. Because sensation is also impaired, caution should be exercised in the use of hot applications.

Mobilising

This may be limited because of cardiac impairment and respiratory distress.

Working and playing

The patient with a radial pulse deficit may be unable to continue in his employment and hobbies.

Sleeping

The patient's normal sleeping pattern may be altered because of some of the physical features of cardiac impairment. Assisting the patient into a fairly upright position with plenty of pillows may help to relieve his discomfort.

Suggested reading

Neutze J, Moller C, Harris E, Horsburgh M, Wilson M 1982 Intensive care of the heart and lungs, 3rd edn. Blackwell Scientific, Oxford, pp 139–173
Nursing Standard 1987 Common arrhythmias. Nursing Standard (Wall chart) 4(2) October 24: 24–25
Roper N, Logan W, Tierney A 1990 The elements of nursing, 3rd edn. Churchill Livingstone, Edinburgh, pp 139–140

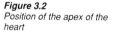

Figure 3.2
Position of the apex of the heart

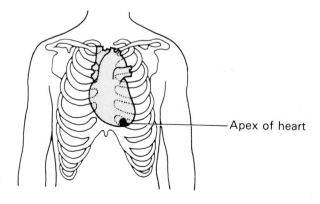

Apex of heart

Blood Pressure

Objectives

By the end of this section you should know how to:

- prepare the patient for this nursing practice
- collect and prepare the equipment
- assess, measure and record blood pressure

Related information

Revision of the anatomy and physiology of the cardiovascular system.

Some indications for the recording of blood pressure

Blood pressure is the force exerted by the blood as it flows through the blood vessels. It is the arterial blood pressure which is normally recorded and this may be indicated:

- to aid in the diagnosis of disease
- to aid in the assessment of the cardiovascular system during and following disease
- preoperatively to assess the patient's usual range of blood pressure
- to aid in assessment of the cardiovascular system following surgery

Equipment

Sphygmomanometer (Fig. 3.3)
Stethoscope

Electronic sphygmomanometers

Increasingly, electronic sphygmomanometers are being used to monitor a patient's blood pressure in general ward areas. Should the nurse encounter any of these machines she should have some instruction on the use of each specific make of sphygmomanometer, as there are variations.

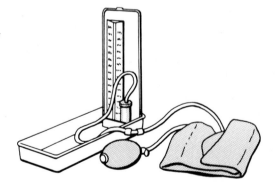

Figure 3.3
Sphygmomanometer: used for blood pressure measurement

Guidelines for this nursing practice

- explain the nursing practice to the patient and gain his consent and cooperation
- wash the hands
- ensure the patient's privacy
- collect the equipment
- observe the patient throughout this activity
- help the patient into a suitable position either sitting or lying and remove restrictive clothing from the arm. Avoid tightly rolled-up sleeves, as this may lead to an inaccurate recording
- position the sphygmomanometer at approximately heart height, ensuring that the mercury level is at zero and the mercury column can be easily read
- apply the cuff 3–5 cm above the point where the brachial artery can be palpated. The cuff should be applied smoothly and firmly with the middle of the rubber bladder directly over the brachial artery
- ask the patient to rest his arm on a suitable firm surface
- connect the cuff tubing to the manometer tubing and close the valve of the inflation ball
- palpate the radial pulse and inflate the cuff until the pulse is obliterated. Inflate a further 20 mmHg. Release the valve slowly taking note of the reading on the mercury column when the radial pulse returns. The mercury is read at the top of the meniscus. Allow all air to escape from the cuff.

- palpate the brachial pulse, place the stethoscope over the site and inflate the cuff to 20 mmHg above the previous reading. Release the valve of the inflation ball at the rate of 2–3 mmHg per second. When the first pulse is heard, the mercury level should be noted. This is the systolic pressure.
- continue to deflate the cuff, and the pulse will change to muffled sounds until finally it disappears; the mercury level should be noted. This is the diastolic pressure
- continue controlled deflation until the point 20 mmHg below the diastolic pressure is reached
- completely deflate the cuff, disconnect the tubing and remove the cuff from the patient's arm
- ensure that the patient is left feeling as comfortable as possible
- if a communal ward stethoscope has been used, clean the ear pieces with an alcohol-saturated swab, to reduce cross-infection between staff
- dispose of the equipment safely
- document the nursing practice appropriately comparing past recordings; note differences, detect trends, monitor after-effects and report abnormal findings immediately

Blood Pressure

Relevance to the activities of living

Maintaining a safe environment

It is recommended that a sphygmomanometer should be calibrated at regular intervals by trained personnel to maintain the accuracy of the equipment.

The size of the cuff is important in achieving accurate recordings. Different sized cuffs are available for use on a baby, child, obese person or recordings on the patient's thigh.

By listening for sounds 20 mmHg above and below the points of appearance and disappearance, the possibility of a 'silent interval' falsifying the reading is overcome.

Repeated measurements, i.e. more than twice in 5 minutes, should be avoided as venous congestion can cause a rise in pressure.

All equipment should be clean and all precautions be taken to prevent cross-infection. The nurse should wash her hands before commencing and on completion of the nursing practice. When a communal ward stethoscope has been used the ear pieces should be cleaned with an alcohol-saturated swab before commencing and on completion of blood pressure assessment. A nurse may wish to purchase her own stethoscope which would prevent any ear cross-infection.

Communicating

Blood pressure measurements can be recorded on a graded chart or abbreviated by placing the systolic pressure reading over the diastolic pressure reading, i.e.

$$\frac{130}{80}$$

Hypertension is the term used when the systolic or diastolic blood pressure is elevated beyond the normal range.

Hypotension is the term used when the blood pressure is lower than the normal range.

Stressful situations of any kind are known to have an effect on a person's blood pressure. When blood pressure recording is part of an admission procedure the nurse should allow the patient to relax before the recording is taken.

Suggested reading

Boore J, Champion R, Ferguson M (eds) 1987 Nursing the physically ill adult. Churchill Livingstone, Edinburgh, pp 611–616

Boylan A, Brown P 1985 The pulse and blood pressure. Nursing Times 81(7) February 13: 26–29

Brunner L, Suddarth D 1988 Textbook of medical–surgical nursing, 6th edn. Lippincott Company, Philadelphia, pp 520–522

Draper P 1987 Not a job for juniors. Nursing Times 83(10) March 11: 58–62 (Recommendations for blood pressure reading)

Faulkner A 1985 Nursing – a creative approach. Baillière Tindall, Eastbourne, pp 172–174

Iveson-Iveson J 1982 Blood pressure. Nursing Mirror 154(12) March 24: 41

Kilgour D, Speedie G 1985 Taking the pressure off. Nursing Mirror 160(9) February 27: 39

O'Brien E, O'Malley K 1979 ABC of blood pressure measurement – the observer. British Medical Journal 2(6193) September 29: 775–776

O'Brien E, O'Malley K 1979 ABC of blood pressure measurement – the sphygmomanometer. British Medical Journal 2(6194) October 6: 851–853

O'Brien E, O'Malley K 1979 ABC of blood pressure measurement – the patient. British Medical Journal 2(6195) October 13: 920–921

O'Brien E, O'Malley K 1979 ABC of blood pressure measurement – the technique. British Medical Journal 2(6196) October 20: 982–984

Roper N, Logan W, Tierney A 1990 The elements of nursing, 3rd edn. Churchill Livingstone, Edinburgh, p 140

Walsh M, Ford P 1989 Nursing rituals – research and rational actions. Heinemann Nursing, Oxford, pp 55–57

Oxygen Therapy

Objectives

By the end of this section you should know how to:

- prepare the patient for this nursing practice
- collect and prepare the equipment
- administer oxygen therapy

Related information

Revision of the anatomy and physiology of the cardiopulmonary system.

Revision of the dangers of the use of oxygen.

Review of health authority policies regarding fire precautions.

Some indications for oxygen therapy

Oxygen therapy is the introduction of increased oxygen to the air available for respiration to prevent hypoxia, a condition where insufficient oxygen is available for the cells of the body, especially those in the brain and vital organs. This may occur in the following circumstances:

- respiratory disease, when the area available for respiration is reduced, e.g.:
  — infection
  — chronic obstructive airways disease (COAD)
  — pulmonary infarction/embolus
  — asthma
- chest injuries following trauma, when the mechanism of respiration may be impaired
- heart disease, when the cardiac output is reduced, e.g.:
  — myocardial infarction
  — congestive cardiac failure

- haemorrhage, when the oxygen-carrying capacity of the blood is reduced
- preoperatively and postoperatively when analgesic drugs may have an effect on respiratory function, e.g. narcotics
- in emergency situations, e.g.:
  — cardiac or respiratory arrest
  — cardiogenic, bacteraemic or haemorrhagic shock

Except in emergency situations oxygen therapy will be prescribed by a medical practitioner, who will specify both the percentage of oxygen and the method of administration.

Equipment

Oxygen supply, e.g. piped oxygen or oxygen cylinder
Reduction gauge as required
Flow meter
Oxygen mask or nasal cannulae as appropriate
Oxygen tubing
Humidifier as appropriate
'No Smoking' signs
Receptacle for soiled disposables

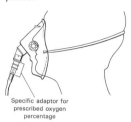

Specific adaptor for
prescribed oxygen
percentage

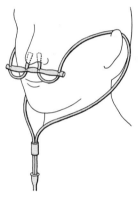

Oxygen masks

Oxygen masks are designed to give an accurate percentage of oxygen by entraining an appropriate amount of air for a specific flow rate of oxygen. Instructions are available for each type of mask and they should be used accordingly.

Edinburgh mask: the percentage of oxygen is adjusted by the flow rate of the flow meter only.

Hudson mask/Venturi mask: with these masks there are various attachments which can be used to give a more specific percentage if prescribed.The required flow of oxygen for the prescribed percentage is given for each attachment, which may be colour coded (Fig. 3.4).

Nasal cannulae

These are light plastic tubes inserted into each nostril, and shaped to fit over the ears to maintain their position. Patients find them less claustrophobic than a conventional mask. They are not suitable for all patients as lower percentages of oxygen are not accurately obtained, and at higher percentages, humidification is inadequate. (Fig. 3.5).

T-piece

Oxygen may be delivered directly into an endotracheal tube or tracheostomy tube via wide corrugated tubing and a T-piece. Adequate humidification is essential.

Oxygen tents

These are used mainly in paediatrics, when babies and young children would not tolerate masks. Danger of fire is increased further using this method, because of the larger area of concentration of oxygen within the oxygen tent, and the difficulty of confining the gas to a small area when nursing the patient.

Emergency situations

For emergency resuscitation procedures, oxygen may be administered via an Ambubag and resuscitation mask (see Cardiopulmonary resuscitation, p. 152).

Humidifiers

It is important that the oxygen administered is adequately humidified to prevent drying of the mucosa of the respiratory tract. There are various humidifiers available.

When percentages of oxygen above 35% are prescribed, humidifiers which nebulise and warm the water vapour should be used, e.g. Inspiron humidifier.

Oxygen Therapy

Guidelines for this nursing practice

- identify and check the prescription for oxygen therapy
- explain the nursing practice to the patient and gain his consent and cooperation
- explain the dangers of smoking to the patient and his visitors and display appropriate 'No Smoking' signs
- collect and assemble the equipment as required
- help the patient into a comfortable position
- observe the patient throughout this activity
- fill the humidifier with sterile water to the correct level
- adjust the flow rate of oxygen as prescribed
- observe the flow of oxygen and water vapour through the mask or cannulae before administration to check that the equipment is working efficiently
- place the mask in the correct position, adjusted to fit firmly and comfortably over the patient's nose and mouth (Fig. 3.4)
- remain with the patient as necessary and help him to maintain the equipment in position
- maintain the level of water in the humidifier as required
- assist the medical practitioner with the estimation of arterial blood gases as required
- observe all precautions to minimise the risk of fire throughout the procedure and while the therapy is still in use
- ensure that the patient is left feeling as comfortable as possible
- dispose of the equipment safely
- document the nursing practice appropriately, monitor after-effects and report abnormal findings immediately

Arterial blood gas estimation

In intensive care areas, accident and emergency units and during perioperative care the effectiveness of oxygen therapy may be monitored by the medical practitioner assessing the arterial blood gases. The results are recorded in relation to the percentage of oxygen administered. Changes in the percentage of oxygen, or methods of administration may be ordered accordingly. Samples of arterial blood are usually obtained from the radial artery, either from an indwelling arterial cannula, or by individual sampling, performed by the medical practitioner. The nurse should maintain observations of the arterial puncture site.

Relevance to the activities of living

Maintaining a safe environment

The patient's general condition should be observed to identify any deterioration or improvement in his hypoxic state, e.g. degree of drowsiness, level of orientation, level of consciousness. The colour and condition of the patient's skin should be observed for the presence of cyanosis, clamminess or sweating.

Oxygen is a gas which readily supports combustion so in areas where it is used, the risk of fire is greatly increased. Every precaution to prevent fire should be maintained. If possible the patient should be aware of the problem and help in maintaining a safe environment, and the dangers of smoking should be explained to him and all his visitors. 'No Smoking' signs can help to reinforce this precaution.

Alcohol-based solutions, oils and grease should not be used in areas where oxygen is administered. These volatile substances are readily flammable and the presence of oxygen will increase the risk of fire.

Health authority policy in association with fire precautions should be familiar to all staff.

The administration of oxygen does not require aseptic technique. However, adequate levels of cleanliness should be maintained to prevent cross-infection, and equipment replaced as necessary. The nurse should wash her hands before commencing and on completion of this nursing practice.

Communicating

Oxygen masks can be a barrier to communication, by making it more difficult for the patient to speak and be heard, so there is a risk of misunderstandings. This may cause the patient to remove the mask. The nurse needs good communication skills, to help the patient tolerate the procedure during the period of time when it is necessary. The use of closed (direct) questions, for which only a 'yes' or 'no' answer is needed, may help with this.

Breathing

In most instances the need for oxygen therapy indicates that the patient has some difficulty with breathing. Dyspnoea may be relieved by helping the patient into an appropriate comfortable position as his condition allows, e.g. sitting upright, leaning over a bed table supported on a pillow, or sitting in a chair.

The respiration rate should be recorded as frequently as necessary, noting the type and depth of the respirations.

Patients who have bronchospasm can be helped by medications which induce bronchodilation, either systematically or via a nebuliser as prescribed (see Nebulisers, p. 94).

Patients who have chronic obstructive airways disease (COAD) have permanently altered respiratory physiology. The respiratory drive or stimulus for respiration only responds to low arterial blood levels of oxygen. Only low percentages of oxygen should be prescribed and administered, e.g. 24%–28% oxygen; raising the arterial blood oxygen level too high in these patients could cause respiratory arrest.

Relevance to the
activities of living
continued

Eating and drinking

The removal of the mask for drinking should be supervised by the nurse, and will depend on the patient's condition.

It may be possible to change to nasal cannulae at meal times only, using a mask at other times to maintain the accuracy of the oxygen percentage as necessary.

Oxygen, even when adequately humidified, causes the mouth and nasal passages to become dry. Frequent oral and nasal hygiene will be required for the patient's comfort, and to maintain a healthy oropharyngeal mucosa.

Personal cleansing and dressing

The patient may need help with both washing and dressing, depending on his condition.

The inside of the oxygen mask may become wet with condensation. The patient's face can be washed and the inside of the mask dried as appropriate. This will greatly increase the patient's comfort and tolerance of this nursing practice.

Expressing sexuality

The use of a face mask has an adverse affect on the patient's self image. The nurse should use good communication skills to counteract this.

Male patients should be helped to shave daily, as this enables the mask to fit comfortably, as well as preserving his self-esteem.

Explanation about the dangers of using perfume or make-up during this procedure should be given to female patients. Extra opportunities for washing and drying the face may help to alleviate the feeling of neglect of her body image.

Suggested reading   Allan D 1989 Making sense of ... oxygen delivery. Nursing Times 85(18) May 3: 40–42
Boore J et al (eds) 1987 Nursing the physically ill adult. Churchill Livingstone, Edinburgh, Ch 24
Cahill C K et al 1990 Sterile water used in low flow oxygen therapy, is it necessary? American Journal of Infection Control 18(1) February 13–17
Campbell J et al 1988 Subjective effects of humidification of oxygen for delivery by nasal cannulae. A prospective study. Chest 93(2) February: 289–293
Roper N, Logan W, Tierney A 1990 The elements of nursing. 3rd edn, Churchill Livingstone, Edinburgh, pp 143–150

Nebulisers

Objectives

By the end of this section you should know how to:

- prepare the patient for this nursing practice
- collect and prepare the equipment
- administer medication via a nebuliser

Related information

Revision of the respiratory system with special reference to respiratory diseases associated with bronchospasm

Revision of oxygen therapy (see p. 88)

Revision of administration of medicines (see p. 12)

Some indications for using nebulisers

A nebuliser attached to a flow of air or oxygen converts a liquid into an aerosol mist which is used as a therapeutic inhalation.

The use of a nebuliser may be indicated for the following reasons:

- to administer bronchodilators for the relief of bronchospasm associated with respiratory disease, e.g.:
  — asthma
  — chronic obstructive airways disease (COAD)
- to administer mucolytic medication to lower the viscosity of the secretions and aid expectoration, e.g.:
  — chronic obstructive airways disease (COAD)
  — cystic fibrosis
  — bronchial carcinoma

The medication, as well as the administration by air or oxygen, is prescribed by a medical practitioner. It may require to be diluted with 2–3 ml normal saline, and is normally prescribed 3–4 times a day. The procedure may be coordinated with chest physiotherapy, and may be administered by a nurse, or the physiotherapist. For the patient with asthma, an estimation of peak flow of tidal volume may be recorded before and after nebuliser therapy.

Equipment

Prescribed air supply; piped, in cylinders, or portable air compressor
Prescribed oxygen supply, either piped or in cylinders
Flow meter
Adaptor
Oxygen tubing
Nebuliser (Fig. 3.6)
Mouthpiece or appropriate oxygen mask, e.g. Hudson mask (Fig. 3.6)
Prescribed medication
Sputum carton as required
'No Smoking' signs as appropriate (see Oxygen therapy, p. 88)
Receptacle for soiled disposables

For peak flow measurement

Peak flow meter
Disposable mouthpiece
Specific chart for documenting results.

Guidelines for this nursing practice

- explain the nursing practice to the patient and gain his consent and cooperation
- ensure the patient's privacy
- prepare and assemble the equipment
- explain the dangers of smoking to the patient and his visitors and position 'No Smoking' signs as appropriate
- help the patient into a comfortable position
- observe the patient throughout the activity
- identify and check the medication prescription (see Administration of medicines, p. 12)
- help the patient to estimate the peak flow of his tidal volume by recording the best of three results on the peak flow meter before commencing nebuliser therapy
- prepare the prescribed dose in a suitable sterile syringe
- fill the nebuliser with prepared medication (Fig. 3.7)
- adjust the flow meter to 5 litres to ensure efficient vaporisation of the medication

- observe the fine spray from the nebuliser to ensure that the equipment is working
- encourage the patient to breathe the nebulised vapour through the mouthpiece for maximum effect; a mask may be used if a patient finds difficulty with the mouthpiece
- remain with the patient until all the solution has been nebulised
- encourage the patient to expectorate
- ensure that the patient is left feeling as comfortable as possible
- help the patient to estimate the peak flow of his tidal volume by recording the best of three results on the peak flow meter. Preferably this should be recorded ½ hr after the completion of nebuliser therapy
- wash and dry the nebuliser, tubing and mask or mouthpiece
- retain the equipment in a polythene bag for the patient's next administration
- document the nursing practice appropriately, monitor after-effects and report abnormal findings immediately

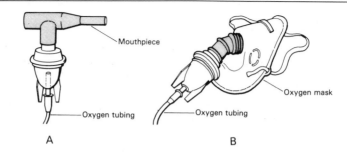

Figure 3.6
Nebuliser
A Attached to a mouthpiece
B Attached to an oxygen
mask

A   B

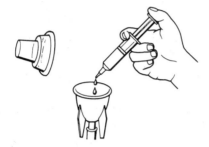

Figure 3.7
Nebuliser taken apart to
introduce a prepared
medication

**Relevance to the
activities of living**

Maintaining a safe environment

If oxygen is used all precautions to prevent the risk of fire should be maintained as with oxygen therapy.

This is not a sterile procedure but adequate standards of cleanliness should be maintained. The nurse should wash her hands before commencing and on completion of this nursing practice.

The equipment for each patient should be kept clean and dry when not in use. It should be changed every 24 hours to prevent infection.

The prescription should be checked by a registered nurse or medical practitioner (see Administration of medicines p. 12).

Communicating

During the nursing practice itself the patient will not be encouraged to speak. Normally all of the solution is administered within 10 minutes and this can be explained to the patient.

Breathing

Monitor the respiration rate, the depth and type of respirations and maintain recordings as frequently as required. The patient should take deep regular breaths through the mouthpiece of the nebuliser to ensure that the medication reaches the mucosa of the bronchi and bronchioles and not just the oropharynx.

Patients will often experience less dyspnoea following this procedure and there may be a dramatic relief of bronchospasm for patients with asthma. This can be monitored by peak flow recordings over a period of time.

Occasionally two drugs are prescribed via the nebuliser and, unless specifically stated, these should *NOT* be mixed. They should be administered in separate nebulisers one after the other, and prescribed bronchodilators should always be administered first. The nebulisers should be labelled appropriately and kept clean and dry for future use.

For efficient vaporisation a flow of 4–5 litres on the flow meter is required. However, for patients with chronic obstructive airways disease this will administer a dangerously high percentage of oxygen (see Oxygen therapy, p. 91) and air should be prescribed for administration instead. This can be a piped supply or in the form of an air compressor.

For patients in intensive care areas a nebuliser can be introduced into the ventilator circuit and medication administered as prescribed.

Observe and record the amount, colour and type of any sputum.

Eating and drinking

A healthy mouth and oropharyngeal mucosa is essential for maximum absorption of the medication. Frequent oral hygiene should be performed as appropriate.

A mouthwash after expectorating may be appreciated and should be available if desired.

Suggested reading

Chilman A, Thomas M 1987 Understanding nursing care, 3rd edn. Churchill Livingstone, Edinburgh, pp 229–240

Ellis P 1990 Asthma: meeting the demand for rapid relief. Professional Nurse 6(2) November: 76, 77, 80, 81

Roper N, Logan W, Tierney A 1990 The elements of nursing, 3rd edn. Churchill Livingstone, Edinburgh, pp 129–149

Smith S 1985 Drugs and the bronchi. Nursing Times 81(7) February 13: 50–51

Steventon R, Wilson R 1986 A guide to apparatus for home nebuliser therapy. Allan & Hanbury. Greenford, pp 3–17

Stokesay J 1989 Breathless. Nursing Times 85(17) April 26: 28–31

Walsh M 1989 Respiration. Asthma, the Orem approach. Nursing 3(38): 18–22

Moist Inhalations

Objectives

By the end of this section you should know how to:

- prepare the patient for this nursing practice
- collect and prepare the equipment
- administer a moist inhalation

Related information

Revision of the respiratory system, with particular reference to respiratory infection.

Revision of administration of medicines (see p. 12).

Review of health authority policy related to moist inhalations.

Some indications for moist inhalations

A moist inhalation involves the inhalation of a medication in warm water, in order to loosen secretions in the upper respiratory tract and promote expectoration. As well as an aid to expectoration, the warm vapour may also ease the pain and discomfort associated with inflammation and frequent coughing.

It is indicated for the following reasons:

- to prevent or treat respiratory infections postoperatively, often in association with physiotherapy
- to treat acute infections of the respiratory tract, e.g. pneumonia, acute bronchitis
- to treat chronic infections of the respiratory tract
- to alleviate the discomfort of patients who have carcinoma of the respiratory tract

Equipment

Nelson steam inhaler or a jug and bowl on a tray, or other commercially prepared equipment
Mouthpiece insulated as appropriate
Boiling water
Large bowl or basin
Insulating cover for inhaler
Towel
Sputum carton
Stable bed table or other appropriate stand
Receptacle for soiled disposables
The inhalation medication which should be prescribed by the medical practitioner, e.g.:
— tincture of benzoin compound
— menthol crystals
Frequency of administration will depend on the patient's condition

Guidelines for this nursing practice

- explain the nursing practice to the patient and gain his consent and cooperation

- prepare and assemble the equipment

- prepare the inhalation medication (prescribed and checked). Note: if menthol is used, one or two crystals are sufficient, and these can be added to the water at the bedside

- cover the inhaler with the insulating cover as appropriate and check that it is at a safe temperature for administration

- help the patient into a comfortable position

- place a towel protectively over the patient's chest

- observe the patient throughout this activity

- place the prepared Nelson steam inhaler on a stable surface with the mouthpiece easily accessible to the patient and the air inlet facing away from the patient (Fig. 3.8)

- encourage the patient to breathe the vapour through his mouth and to breathe out through his nose

- remain with the patient for the duration of the practice and observe his condition. Note: the effectiveness of the inhalation will last for approximately 10 minutes

- help the patient to cough and expectorate as appropriate

- ensure that the patient is left feeling as comfortable as possible

- dispose of the equipment safely

- document the nursing practice appropriately, monitor after-effects and report abnormal findings immediately

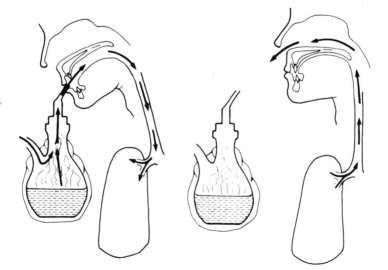

Figure 3.8
Moist inhalation using a Nelson's inhaler: inhaling through the mouth and exhaling through the nasal passage (Reproduced with permission from Roper N, Logan W, Tierney A 1985 The elements of nursing, 2nd edn. Churchill Livingstone, Edinburgh)

Relevance to the activities of living

Maintaining a safe environment

During the preparation and administration every precaution should be taken to prevent the risk of scalding when handling the hot water and when in contact with the hot vapour.

The equipment should be washed and dried between administrations, and kept for the one patient during the period of treatment, to limit the risk of cross-infection. The nurse should wash her hands before commencing and on completion of the nursing practice.

In order to maintain a safe environment inhalations should only be administered to patients who are fully conscious and well orientated. The full cooperation of the patient is needed for maximum effectiveness of the inhalation and for the safety of the procedure.

The nurse should remain with the patient during this nursing practice.

Communicating

Occasionally this practice is prescribed to alleviate pain and discomfort associated with respiratory disease. For patients with carcinoma of the respiratory system it can have a very helpful psychological effect when used with other means of pain relief as required.

Breathing

The pulse and respiratory rates should be monitored, especially the rate and depth of respirations. This practice will normally be prescribed for patients with respiratory disease but all other nursing care for the relief of dyspnoea should be maintained as appropriate.

If the practice is prescribed to aid expectoration it can be scheduled to coincide with chest physiotherapy in cooperation with the physiotherapist. The nurse should encourage the patient to cough and expectorate at other times, in between treatments, and the colour and type of sputum should be noted.

Eating and drinking

To maintain a healthy oral mucosa, oral hygiene should be performed as frequently as necessary. A mouthwash after expectorating may be appreciated by the patient and should be available if desired.

Sleeping

To help the patient to be as comfortable as possible and so induce sleep, it may be helpful for the last administration of inhalation to be given before settling for the night.

Suggested reading   Chilman A, Thomas M 1987 Understanding nursing care, 3rd edn. Churchill
                          Livingstone, Edinburgh, pp 229–240
                          Roper N, Logan W, Tierney A 1990 The elements of nursing. 3rd edn, Churchill
                          Livingstone, Edinburgh, pp 139–149

Specimen of Sputum

Objectives

By the end of this section you should know how to:

- prepare the patient for this nursing practice
- obtain from a patient a specimen of sputum for examination

Related information

Revision of the anatomy and physiology of the respiratory system.

Some indications for collecting a specimen of sputum

Sputum results from an excessive production of mucus in the respiratory tract.

A specimen may be required:

- to observe the colour and consistency as an aid to the diagnosis of disease and to monitor the effect of treatment
- to permit laboratory culture, to identify pathogenic microorganisms and

determine drug sensitivity

- to permit cytological examination as an aid to the diagnosis of disease

Equipment

Sterile glass or plastic container with lid, appropriately labelled
Laboratory form
Plastic specimen bag for transportation

Guidelines for this nursing practice

- explain the nursing practice to the patient and gain his consent and cooperation
- ensure the patient's privacy
- collect the specimen in the early morning if possible, before food or fluid has been taken by the patient which might mix with the specimen
- ensure that no antiseptic mouthwash or toothpaste has been used prior to collection as this may alter the bacteriological count
- encourage the patient to cough the material from the lungs, by deep breathing several times, then coughing vigorously and expectorating into the container

- avoid contamination by the sputum of the hands of the nurse or patient, or the outside of the container
- ensure the patient is left feeling as comfortable as possible
- dispatch the labelled specimen container immediately to the laboratory with the completed form
- document this nursing practice appropriately, monitor after-effects and report abnormal findings immediately

Relevance to the activities of living

Maintaining a safe environment

For the safe transport of specimens see Specimen collection (p. 198).

Breathing

If the patient has difficulty expectorating, the physiotherapist may, with appropriate exercises, help the patient to cough, loosen mucus and produce sputum.

Personal cleansing and dressing

The patient may appreciate a mouthwash after expectorating, and this should be offered following the specimen collection.

Expressing sexuality

The patient may find it embarrassing to spit into a container. A clear explanation of the reason for the specimen should be given to the patient and he should be allowed as much privacy as possible.

Suggested reading

Ayton M 1982 Microbiological investigations. Nursing 2 (8) December: 226
Hamilton H (ed) 1985 Nurse's reference library – procedures. Springhouse Corporation, Pennsylvania, pp 483–492
Keane C (ed) 1986 Essentials of medical–surgical nursing. W.B. Saunders, Philadelphia, p 304
Roper N, Logan W, Tierney A 1990 The elements of nursing, 3rd edn. Churchill Livingstone, Edinburgh, pp 145–146

Intravenous Infusion

There are four parts to this section:

1 **Commencing an intravenous infusion**
2 **Priming the equipment for intravenous infusion**
3 **Maintaining the infusion for a period of time**
4 **Venepuncture**

The concluding subsection, 'Relevance to the activities of living', refers to all four practices collectively.

Objectives

By the end of this section you should know how to:

- prepare the patient for these nursing practices
- collect and prepare the equipment
- assist the medical practitioner with the safe insertion of an intravenous cannula
- maintain an intravenous infusion as prescribed

Related information

Revision of the anatomy and physiology of the cardiovascular system, with special reference to the circulation of the blood, and body fluids.

Revision of aseptic technique (see p. 26).

Review of health authority policy in relation to intravenous therapy.

Some indications for intravenous infusion

An intravenous infusion is the introduction of prescribed sterile fluid into the blood circulation and may be indicated for the following reasons:

- to maintain a normal fluid, nutrient and electrolyte balance when the patient is unable to maintain adequate intake by mouth, and nasogastric feeding is inappropriate, e.g.:
  — a patient during the preoperative and postoperative period
  — a patient who has had surgery involving the alimentary system
  — a patient who has malabsorption problems

- to replace severe fluid loss in emergency situations, e.g.:
  — a patient who has severe haemorrhage and haemorrhagic shock
  — a patient who has severe burns or scalds
  — a patient dehydrated by vomiting or diarrhoea usually associated with enteric infection

- to administer medication when other routes are not appropriate, e.g.:
  — analgesic medication for effective pain relief
  — anticoagulant therapy for treatment of deep vein thrombosis

1 COMMENCING AN INTRAVENOUS INFUSION

Outline of the procedure

Intravenous therapy is prescribed and initiated by the medical practitioner using aseptic technique. The nurse may be required to help with the procedure, to safely maintain the infusion for a period of time, and to help with the removal of the cannula.

Using aseptic technique the medical practitioner chooses a suitable vein site for access, the skin area is shaved as necessary and cleansed with antiseptic lotion. A local anaesthetic may be injected around the vein site if required. A sterile cannula is inserted into the vein so that the prescribed infusion fluid can enter the patient's blood circulation. The infusion fluid flows into the cannula through an administration set which will have been primed ready for use. The cannula is secured in position and covered by a sterile dressing. The flow of infusion fluid is maintained, and the containers of fluid replaced as prescribed until the intravenous infusion is discontinued.

Sites chosen for intravenous cannulation

Short-term intravenous therapy: The veins at the back of the hand or the superficial veins of the wrist or lower arm are chosen for short-term infusions expected to last hours or a few days. Cannulation increases the risk of venous thrombosis in the veins used for access; if this occurs in the smaller branches of peripheral veins following an infusion, it is still possible to use the larger branches of the same vein at a later date if required. Veins of the lower limbs are rarely used because of the increased risk of thrombosis, due to a slower venous flow. To minimise the patient's discomfort the non-dominant limb should be used if possible.

Long-term intravenous therapy: For long-term intravenous infusions lasting several days or weeks, a long catheter is inserted into the subclavian vein or the internal jugular vein so that the tip of the catheter lies in the superior vena cava (see Parenteral nutrition, p. 174; Central venous pressure, p. 124).

Equipment

Trolley
Sterile dressings pack
Sterile cannula as required by the medical practitioner
Alcohol-based antiseptic for cleansing the skin
Sterile administration set
Prescribed sterile infusion fluid
Sterile transparent dressing
Infusion stand
Tourniquet or sphygmomanometer
Hypoallergenic tape
Receptacle for soiled disposables

Equipment
continued

Additional equipment if required

Equipment for shaving the skin area

Local anaesthetic and equipment for its administration

Air inlet for glass containers

Holder for glass containers (bottle holder)

Splint and bandage to support the limb where the infusion is sited

Continuous infusion pump and appropriate cassette (see Parenteral nutrition, p. 174)

Infusion fluids

The most commonly prescribed fluids are:
— normal saline (sodium chloride 0.9%)
— dextrose 5% in water
— Ringer's Lactate
— plasma or plasma expanders, e.g. Haemaccel, stable plasma protein solution (SPPS)
— blood (see Blood transfusion, p. 118)
— parenteral nutrients (see Parenteral nutrition, p. 174).

Most prescribed fluids are commercially prepared in sterile containers and they are labelled FOR INTRAVENOUS INFUSION. They may also be prepared by the hospital pharmacy. The containers used for these preparations are frequently soft plastic bags protected by an outer covering (see manufacturer's instructions), although glass bottles or semi-rigid plastic containers (Polyfusors) continue to be used for some preparations.

Cannulae

Various cannulae (Fig. 3.9) are available, and are prepared commercially in sterile packs. Those chosen by the medical practitioner may have an inner needle surrounded by a plastic cannula. The needle is withdrawn once the vein is punctured, allowing blood to flow back. Once the cannula is safely in situ the infusion fluid is connected and the cannula is secured in position. Some cannula packs include an accompanying syringe, e.g. Medicut. Small winged needles are used for access to scalp veins in babies and young children.

Figure 3.9
*Intravenous infusion:
cannulae in common use
A Cannula used when
intravenous drugs are to be
administered with the infusion
or post-infusion
B Cannula used
preoperatively for short-term
infusion*

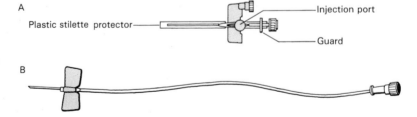

A

Plastic stilette protector

Injection port

Guard

B

Administration sets

Administration sets are commercially prepared in sterile packs. The set contains specialised sterile tubing; at one end there is a rigid trocar protected by a sterile sheath. At the other end is a similarly protected Luer connector nozzle. Towards the trocar end, the tubing widens into a drip chamber. An adjustable roller clamp surrounds the tubing below the drip chamber, which allows the flow of fluid to be regulated for the prescribed flow rate. Blood administration sets include a filter. Simple administration sets are available without filter, for infusion of clear fluids (Fig. 3.10).

Figure 3.10
Administration set for intravenous infusion

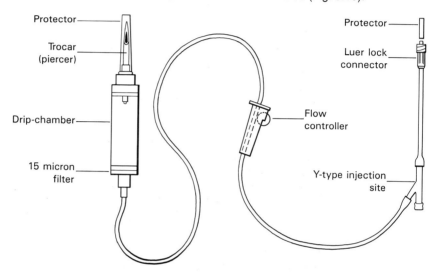

Specialised administration sets (burette set)

A specialised administration set is used for infusions when a volumetric infusion pump is not available and a more accurate control of flow rate is needed. This is particularly important when infusions are prescribed for babies or young children to reduce the risk of fluid overload. The burette set has a calibrated drip chamber, with one roller clamp above and one roller clamp below. The drip chamber is filled with the amount of fluid prescribed in ml per hour. This amount of fluid is infused during one hour. The flow rate will depend on the drop factor and the amount prescribed (see manufacturer's instructions). In order for the infusion to continue, the drip chamber has to be refilled as prescribed each time it is emptied.

Volumetric infusion pumps

Volumetric infusion pumps are used with specific sterile cassettes (e.g. Accuset) as well as a normal administration set so that an accurate flow of fluid can be maintained during the infusion (see manufacturer's instructions). When primed and connected these can be set to infuse fluid within a range of 1–999 ml per hour. This equipment is expensive and is used extensively in intensive care areas but only occasionally in the general wards, mainly for the administration of intravenous medication or parenteral nutrition (see Parenteral nutrition, p. 174).

Syringe pumps may be used for a continuous infusion of prescribed intravenous medication of less than 10 ml per hour.

Guidelines for this nursing practice

- help to explain the nursing practice to the patient and gain his consent and cooperation
- ensure the patient's privacy
- help to collect and prepare the equipment
- check the prescribed infusion fluid with a registered nurse or medical practitioner
- prime the administration set with the infusion fluid maintaining asepsis
- place the infusion fluid on the stand beside the patient, check that it is running freely and all air is expelled from the system. The end should be protected by replacing the sterile cap if not connected immediately
- help the patient into as comfortable a position as possible
- observe the patient throughout this activity
- expose and support the area for cannulation

- help to prepare the sterile equipment as required
- apply pressure around the limb above the cannulation site as directed using a sphygmomanometer cuff or tourniquet. This will maintain more blood in the veins and facilitate cannulation
- release the pressure as directed once the venous cannula is correctly positioned, and the infusion lines are connected
- regulate the flow rate as prescribed
- help the medical practitioner to secure the dressing and tubing (Fig. 3.11)
- apply a splint to the limb if appropriate
- ensure that the patient is left feeling as comfortable as possible
- document this nursing practice appropriately, monitor after-effects and report abnormal findings immediately
- maintain the infusion at the prescribed flow rate

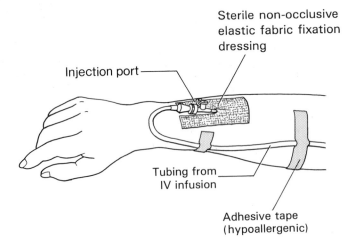

Figure 3.11
Intravenous infusion: anchoring the tubing with adhesive tape

Sterile non-occlusive elastic fabric fixation dressing

Injection port

Tubing from IV infusion

Adhesive tape (hypoallergenic)

2 PRIMING THE EQUIPMENT FOR INTRAVENOUS INFUSION

This is the preparation of the prescribed infusion fluid by running it through the administration set. Asepsis should be maintained during this part of the practice to prevent any internal or exposed areas being contaminated.

Equipment

Prescribed intravenous infusion fluid
Sterile administration set
Sterile gallipot
Receptacle for soiled disposables
Infusion stand
Alcohol-saturated swab
Sterile air inlet }
Bottle holder   } for use with glass container
Trolley or tray

Guidelines for this nursing practice

- check the infusion fluid which is prescribed by the medical practitioner. Each container of fluid is checked by two people, one of whom must be a registered nurse or a medical practitioner (see Administration of medicines, p. 12)
- check the following details against the patient's own documentation and the label on the infusion fluid:
  — the patient's name and unit number
  — the date of the prescription
  — the type of infusion prescribed
  — the amount of infusion prescribed
  — the container labelled 'for intravenous infusion'
  — the expiry date of the infusion fluid
  — the time prescribed for commencement of the infusion
  — the time to be taken for completion of the infusion
  — the signature of the medical practitioner

- check the fluid for cloudiness, sediment or discoloration. The container should be checked for any flaws, leaks or evidence of contamination. Any suspect fluid or containers must be discarded immediately according to health authority policies
- include the serial number of the fluid as well as the signature of the nurse or medical practitioner checking the infusion prescription in the documentation
- establish the identity of the patient by appropriate means, e.g. identification bracelet

Guidelines for this nursing practice *continued*

When using a soft plastic container (bag):

- perform appropriate hand washing technique
- remove the outer plastic covering of the container
- remove the sheath covering the entry channel, without contaminating the inside
- remove the administration set from its package
- close the flow control clamp
- remove the protective sheath from the trocar of the administration set, maintaining asepsis
- insert the trocar firmly through the seal of the container's entry channel until fluid flows into the first part of the administration set
- invert the container and hang it on the infusion pole
- gently squeeze the chamber of the administration set and allow it to partly fill

- temporarily remove the protective sheath covering the Luer connector at the end of the administration set, holding it clear of any contamination, preferably over a sterile container (e.g. gallipot)
- slowly release the flow control clamp and allow the fluid to fill the rest of the tubing
- eliminate any air bubbles from the fluid in the tubing, by running some fluid into a sterile container if necessary
- close the flow control clamp
- replace the protective cover on the Luer connector nozzle
- place the free end of the tubing in the notch provided on the flow control clamp, keeping the Luer connector nozzle protected from contamination
- place the primed equipment on the infusion stand beside the patient's bed ready for connection to the intravenous cannula

The equipment should only be primed immediately prior to the infusion to minimise the risk of infection.

If contamination occurs or the container is punctured while priming the equipment, the infusion and the administration set are discarded and the procedure recommenced.

When using a glass container (bottle):

- maintain aseptic technique as before
- remove the seal from the top of the checked infusion fluid bottle
- clean the rubber bung with alcohol solution
- prepare the administration set as before
- push the trocar firmly through the rubber bung
- remove the sterile air inlet from its outer package and remove the protective sheath from the needle

- insert the needle of the air inlet through the rubber bung
- hang the inverted bottle on the infusion stand using a bottle holder if required and support the end of the air inlet above the level of the fluid in the bottle if necessary
- proceed to prime the equipment as before

When using a semi-rigid plastic container (Polyfusor):

- maintain aseptic technique as before
- remove the outer package of the checked infusion fluid
- cut off the end of the entry channel with sterile scissors to maintain asepsis
- prepare the administration set as before

- insert the trocar into the entry channel and twist it for a firm fit
- invert the container and hang it on the infusion stand
- proceed to prime the equipment as before (no air inlet is required for this container)

3   MAINTAINING THE INFUSION FOR A PERIOD OF TIME

In order to maintain the flow of infusion at the prescribed rate, the number of drops per minute required for each particular infusion has to be accurately calculated.

Guidelines for this nursing practice

Calculating the flow rate of infusion fluids

All administration sets include details of the number of drops per ml for that particular set. This is known as the drop factor. Some sets include a scale of drops per minute for a given time within the pack.

Formula used for calculation

$$\frac{\text{Total volume of infusion fluid} \times \text{Drop factor (see administration set)}}{\text{Total time of infusion in minutes}}$$

Example

Total volume of fluid   = 500 ml

Time for completion   = 4 hours, i.e. 240 minutes (4×60)

Drop factor   = 15

$$\frac{500 \times 15}{240} = 31.2 = 30 \text{ drops (approx)}$$

Thus the number of drops required to maintain the infusion at the required rate = 30 per minute when drop factor is 15 drops per ml.

The position of the cannula in the vein and the movement of the patient's limbs may have an effect on the flow rate. It is important to visually assess the rate of fall of fluid in the infusion container as well as to regulate the required drops per minute, e.g. when the time for completion is 4 hours, one quarter of the fluid should have been infused after 1 hour, and half the fluid after 2 hours.

Changing the infusion container

Within 24 hours the empty container can be replaced with a full container of prescribed infusion fluid without changing the administration set. The containers should be exchanged before the level of fluid drops below the point of the trocar in the neck of the container. Preparation for changing a container should begin while a small amount of fluid remains in the infusion container; this prevents the formation of air bubbles in the system and the danger of air embolus.

Intravenous Infusion

Guidelines for this
nursing practice
continued

- explain the nursing practice to the patient and gain his consent and cooperation
- perform hand washing and maintain asepsis during this practice as before
- check the prescribed infusion fluid
- prepare the new container of infusion fluid as for priming the equipment
- turn off the infusion temporarily, by closing the roller clamp
- remove the trocar of the administration set from the empty container and insert it into the new infusion fluid, maintaining asepsis (a new air inlet should be used when changing glass bottles)

- recommence the infusion as soon as possible at the prescribed flow rate
- maintain observations as before
- dispose of the used container safely
- document the nursing practice appropriately, monitor after-effects and report abnormal findings immediately

Removal of the intravenous cannula

This is performed using aseptic technique when an intravenous infusion is discontinued or when a new site for access is needed for continuing an infusion.

- explain the procedure to the patient and obtain his consent and cooperation
- ensure the patient's privacy
- close the flow clamp to discontinue infusion of fluid
- prepare a trolley and sterile dressings as required
- don sterile gloves to prevent blood-borne cross-infection
- expose the site of insertion of the cannula, maintaining asepsis
- remove retaining sutures if present (see p. 31)
- apply pressure with a sterile swab using the non-dominant hand, and withdraw the cannula slowly with the dominant hand, maintaining pressure

- retain pressure on the puncture site as required until bleeding stops, maintaining asepsis
- cover the site with a small sterile dressing, e.g. Airstrip
- dispose of equipment safely
- resume observation of the site as appropriate
- document the nursing practice appropriately, monitor after-effects and report abnormal findings immediately

Occasionally the tip of the cannula is sent to the laboratory for microbiological investigation. If this is ordered the tip is cut off with sterile scissors, put into an appropriately labelled sterile specimen container, maintaining asepsis, and sent to the appropriate laboratory with the completed laboratory form (see Specimen collection, p. 198).

4 VENEPUNCTURE

In the UK this is performed by the medical practitioner either to obtain a sample of blood for investigation, or to administer intravenous medication. In special care units, and in the community, this may be performed by qualified nursing staff. Normally a needle connected to a syringe is used for access to a vein, maintaining aseptic technique. The nurse should inspect any venepuncture site for leakage, infection or bruising. Occasionally a small specialised cannula is inserted into a vein and left in situ for a few hours, or several days. Intravenous medication may be administered, or samples of blood removed. Observations of the site and cannula should be maintained and any abnormalities reported as for intravenous infusion.

Relevance to the activities of living

Maintaining a safe environment

Intravenous infusion is an invasive practice so all precautions must be maintained to prevent any infection occurring at the venous access site, or infection entering the blood circulation via the infusion itself (Fig. 3.12). Efficient hand washing technique should be employed when handling equipment.

Figure 3.12
Potential routes for contamination associated with intravenous infusion

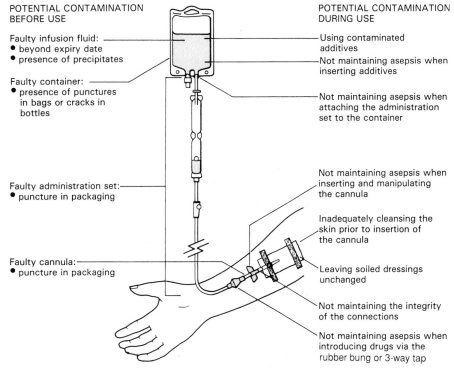

POTENTIAL CONTAMINATION BEFORE USE

Faulty infusion fluid:
• beyond expiry date
• presence of precipitates

Faulty container:
• presence of punctures in bags or cracks in bottles

Faulty administration set:
• puncture in packaging

Faulty cannula:
• puncture in packaging

POTENTIAL CONTAMINATION DURING USE

Using contaminated additives

Not maintaining asepsis when inserting additives

Not maintaining asepsis when attaching the administration set to the container

Not maintaining asepsis when inserting and manipulating the cannula

Inadequately cleansing the skin prior to insertion of the cannula

Leaving soiled dressings unchanged

Not maintaining the integrity of the connections

Not maintaining asepsis when introducing drugs via the rubber bung or 3-way tap

Relevance to the
activities of living
continued

The drip rate and the flow rate should be monitored to check that there is no occlusion in the system, and that the prescribed flow is maintained. Spasm of the vein or movement of the limb may cause slowing or stopping of the infusion and repositioning the limb may help to relieve the occlusion. If the stoppage is associated with soreness or swelling of the vein site this may indicate that the cannula is no longer in the vein and fluid is seeping into the surrounding tissues, or be evidence of developing thrombophlebitis. If this occurs the medical practitioner should be informed, the infusion discontinued and replaced at another site.

All the equipment connections should be inspected for any disconnections, flaws or leakage, to prevent contamination or the possibility of an air embolus. The tubing should be inspected to check that there are no air bubbles.

Careful, considerate explanation of what the practice involves will help the patient to cooperate in maintaining a safe environment. He should understand the reasons why the lines must not be pulled or the dressing touched.

Patients who are confused or disorientated may require the appropriate use of splints and bandages to safely maintain the infusion in position.

The administration set should be changed every 24 hours, maintaining asepsis to minimise the risk of infection, unless long term (96 hour) filters are used.

The dressing should be changed according to local practice. A transparent sterile occlusive dressing enables the site and the cannula to be observed without disturbing the dressing, and this can minimise the risk of infection. Gloves should be worn to prevent the risk of blood-borne infection.

Any abnormalities should be reported immediately and the infusion discontinued, or the rate of infusion reduced to a minimum until further instructions are given. Maintaining minimum flow will prevent clotting in the vein and also reduce the risk of further complications developing until the problem has been dealt with.

Communicating

The patient may find this practice very stressful, and the nurse should give appropriate support, and simple explanations at each stage of the procedure.

It may be difficult for the patient to position spectacles or a hearing aid if one hand is immobilised. By anticipating his needs the nurse can greatly enhance the patient's ability to communicate. He should be reassured that a nurse is always nearby and constantly observant. When leaving the patient the nurse should ensure that articles he is likely to need are easily accessible and that a bell or other means of communication is available.

Breathing

Intravenous therapy in itself should not affect the patient's breathing but vital signs should be monitored hourly, 2-hourly or 4-hourly according to circumstances so that complications can be identified as soon as possible.

The pulse rate: Tachycardia may indicate infusion reaction or infection. It may also indicate circulatory overload if the rate of infusion is too rapid and the patient's cardiac output has difficulty in responding to the extra fluid in the circulation.

The respiration rate: A rise in respiration rate may indicate infection or circulatory overload. Dyspnoea accompanied by a cough and frothy sputum may indicate pulmonary oedema and should be reported immediately.

The blood pressure: Changes in blood pressure will depend on the reason for infusion. If the infusion is given to replace fluid loss, the patient may be hypotensive initially and a gradual rise in blood pressure will be expected. Recordings outside the normal range should be reported.

The prescribed rate of the infusion will depend on the individual patient's requirements and condition. Patients who have congestive cardiac failure and elderly patients will have a lower infusion rate prescribed by the medical practitioner.

The prescribed rate of infusion for babies and young children will be adjusted for their age, weight and height ratio. A volumetric infusion pump or a burette set should be used to maintain an accurate flow rate, and observations monitored frequently.

For seriously ill patients a catheter may be inserted to record the central venous pressure, which can accurately monitor changes in circulating fluid volume during the period of intravenous infusion (see Central venous pressure, p. 124).

Disconnection of the infusion lines may cause a backflow of blood, increasing the risk of haemorrhage. Pressure over the venous site will prevent further blood loss, while appropriate action is taken by qualified staff.

An air embolus may occur if a bubble of air enters the blood circulation. The bubble may remain unnoticed until it reaches the heart. A large air embolus may cause a cardiac arrest; a small one may enter the pulmonary circulation and cause some respiratory distress. Every effort should be made to eliminate air from the tubing when priming the infusion equipment, and observations maintained to prevent any risk of air embolus occurring (see Central venous pressure, p. 124).

Eating and drinking

Fluid intake should be recorded and fluid balance charts accurately maintained.

Normally the amount of infusion fluid is documented after the completion of each unit. However, with seriously ill patients both intake and output are recorded hourly. In this case the infusion fluid is usually given via continuous infusion pump or a burette set.

The patient may be unable to eat or drink normally during this procedure. Oral hygiene should be performed as appropriate to maintain a healthy oral and oropharyngeal mucosa (see Mouth care, p. 268).

The infusion may continue during the period of time when the patient recommences oral feeding. The food should be prepared so that the patient can comfortably use his available hand and the nurse should ensure that prescribed oral fluids are readily accessible if one arm is partly immobilised by the infusion equipment.

Eliminating

Accurate documentation of fluid output should be maintained. This will help to monitor the patient's renal function during the infusion.

The patient may need help when using a commode, to support the administration lines and prevent disconnection of tubing.

Relevance to the
activities of living
continued

Personal cleansing and dressing

The condition of the skin should be noted. Local redness or heat may indicate infection, and swelling may indicate fluid leakage into the surrounding tissues; sweating, shivering, rigor, pallor or a rash may indicate an adverse systemic reaction (see pharmaceutical literature).

The patient may need appropriate help with personal cleansing and dressing.

Clothing may have to be adapted to maintain access to the infusion site. The need for this and appropriate light clothing should be explained to the patient.

Controlling body temperature

Body temperature should be monitored hourly, 2-hourly or 4-hourly according to circumstances. A sudden rise in body temperature, or shivering and signs of rigor, may indicate infusion reaction or the onset of infection and should be reported immediately (see Blood transfusion, p. 118).

It may be necessary for the area of the infusion site to be exposed for observation. The patient may need help to adjust his own clothing, or the bedcovers, for any perceived change in temperature.

Mobilising

Increasingly, patients are encouraged to move around and even to take a shower as their condition allows while an intravenous infusion is still in progress, especially during the postoperative period. The nurse should ensure that the lines are supported and all precautions for prevention of infection and disconnection are maintained with the patient's cooperation, during the period of mobilising.

Working and playing

The nurse should ensure that the patient maintains his interests, as his condition allows, while this practice is in progress. Access to newspapers, radio and television should be available if required.

Families and friends should be encouraged to visit the patient if there are no other contraindications.

Sleeping

The patient's general condition should be noted, e.g. restlessness, drowsiness and level of consciousness.

The patient may find it difficult to lie in his normal sleeping position due to the infusion. Help in adjusting to a suitably comfortable position may induce sleep.

Necessary observations may waken the patient. Explanation of the need for these and reassurance may reduce the waking period. The observations which cause the most disturbance are the recording of temperature and blood pressure. These observations may be reduced in frequency as the patient's condition allows, while maintaining the frequency of the pulse rate recording and observations of the lines and infusion rate.

Suggested reading

Boore J et al (eds) 1987 Nursing the physically ill adult. Churchill Livingstone, Edinburgh, pp 838–842

Fincham Gee C, Noble W 1990 Transparent film dressings. Nursing 4(21) October 25: 39–41

Goodison S M 1990 Keeping the flora out. Professional Nurse 5(11) August: 572–575

Heckler J 1988 Improved techniques in IV therapy. Nursing Times 84(34) August 24: 28–33

Krakowska G 1986 Nursing practice versus procedure. Nursing Times 82(40) December 3: 64–69

Mulhan D A 1988 Managing complications of IV therapy. Nursing 3(18) March: 34–42

Roper N, Logan W, Tierney A 1990 The elements of nursing. 3rd edn. Churchill Livingstone, Edinburgh, pp 136–142

Sadler C 1989 How nurses help children cope with a Hickman catheter. Nursing 3(47) December 7: 30–31

Speechley V et al 1989 Managing an implantable drug delivery system (port-a-cath). Professional Nurse 4(6) March: 284–5, 287–8

Walsh M, Ford P 1989 Nursing rituals, research and rational actions. Heinemann Nursing, Oxford pp 21–25

Blood Transfusion

Objectives

By the end of this section you should know how to:

- prepare the patient for this nursing practice
- collect and prepare equipment
- assist the medical practitioner with the safe insertion of an intravenous cannula
- maintain a blood transfusion for a period of time

Related information

Revision of the anatomy and physiology of the blood, with special emphasis on blood groups.

Revision of intravenous therapy (see p. 104).

Revision of aseptic technique (see p. 26).

Review of health authority policy in relation to blood transfusion.

Some indications for a blood transfusion

A blood transfusion is the introduction of prepared compatible donor blood into the circulation of a recipient patient. A blood transfusion may be indicated for the following reasons:

- to restore circulatory blood volume following haemorrhage
- to maintain adequate circulatory blood volume during and following surgical procedures
- to maintain adequate haemoglobin levels which have been reduced by blood disorders, e.g. anaemia, leukaemia

Blood for transfusion is prescribed and ordered by a medical practitioner.

Blood is cross-matched in the blood transfusion laboratory for compatibility, to correspond with the blood group of the individual recipient, and labelled accordingly.

Each unit of blood ordered is stored in the blood bank at 1–6°C for use within 48 hours.

Equipment

As for intravenous infusion

Additional equipment

Grouped and cross-matched unit of prescribed blood
Sterile blood administration set
Sterile blood filter as appropriate
Non-sterile gloves which should be worn when handling all blood products

In emergency situations

Pressure bag (Fenwal bag)
Blood warming equipment

Guidelines for this nursing practice

This procedure will be initiated by a medical practitioner using aseptic technique. Blood should be transfused by a separate intravenous route from all other infusions. This may necessitate a separate peripheral intravenous line for the duration of the blood transfusion only (see Intravenous therapy, p. 104).

- help to explain the nursing practice to the patient and gain his consent and cooperation

- ensure the patient's privacy

- collect and prepare the equipment

- help the patient into a comfortable position as required

- observe the patient throughout this activity

- obtain the prescribed unit of blood from the blood bank immediately prior to use

- check that the blood is compatible for that particular patient

- prime the administration set with normal saline (Fig. 3.13). Note: only normal saline (sodium chloride 0.9%) is compatible with blood and no other IV fluid should be used

- assist the medical practitioner as required with the insertion of an intravenous cannula (see intravenous therapy p. 104)

- commence the transfusion of blood at the prescribed rate

- help the patient into a comfortable position following the commencement of the transfusion

- maintain the flow of blood at the prescribed rate

- record accurately the volume of blood transfused. Note: the volume of one unit of whole blood is 500 ml: the volume of one unit of concentrated red cells is 300 ml

- ensure that the patient is left feeling as comfortable as possible

- dispose of the equipment safely

- document this nursing practice appropriately, monitor after-effects, and report abnormal findings immediately

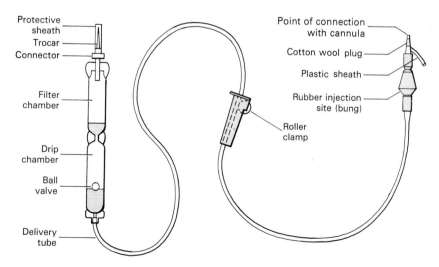

Figure 3.13
Administration set for blood transfusion. An extra filter may be introduced between the blood pack and the blood administration set

Protective sheath
Trocar
Connector
Filter chamber
Drip chamber
Ball valve
Delivery tube

Point of connection with cannula
Cotton wool plug
Plastic sheath
Rubber injection site (bung)
Roller clamp

Blood Transfusion

Guidelines for this
nursing practice
continued

Guidelines for withdrawal of blood from the bank

- refer to health authority policies for access to the blood bank and local procedure

- withdraw blood from the blood bank one unit at a time immediately before transfusion for an individual patient

- check information on the label of the blood container against appropriate documentation for that particular patient

- complete documentation of withdrawal for the blood transfusion service and the patient's medical records

Guidelines for checking blood for transfusion

Blood for transfusion is checked by two people, one of whom must be a medical practitioner or a registered nurse.

- identify the prescription for blood transfusion and check the following information:
  — the date and time of commencement
  — the name of the patient
  — the unit or hospital number of the patient
  — the type of blood prescribed, e.g. whole blood or concentrated red cells
  — the number of units prescribed
  — the rate of transfusion ordered
  — the signature of the medical practitioner

- check the following information against the patient's own documentation and each labelled unit of blood:
  — the name of the patient
  — the unit or hospital number of the patient
  — the age and date of birth of the patient
  — the address of the patient
  — the blood group of the patient
  — the rhesus factor of the patient
  — the expiry date of the blood pack
  — the unit number of the blood pack

- establish the patient's identity by appropriate means, e.g. identification bracelet

- sign the label on the checked blood unit; this is signed by the two people involved

- transfer the duplicate unit pack number to the patient's records according to health authority policy

Relevance to the activities of living

Maintaining a safe environment

Gloves should be worn at all times when handling blood products and associated equipment to prevent cross-infection from blood-borne viral infections such as hepatitis B or HIV AIDS and to protect staff from invasive contact (see Isolation nursing, p. 36).

All precautions for the prevention of infection and the prevention of air emboli should be maintained (see Intravenous infusion, p. 104).

Accurate checking of individual units of blood will help to ensure that only compatible blood is transfused.

Despite careful cross-matching some patients develop a transfusion reaction, but accurate observations will help to detect this as early as possible. All observations should be continued for at least 4 hours after the last unit of blood has been transfused, and thereafter as appropriate.

If a transfusion reaction is suspected, the transfusion is discontinued and the medical practitioner informed immediately. The haematologist should also be informed, and used blood containers returned to the blood transfusion laboratory for testing.

Communicating

Any complaint of pain should be reported, e.g. headache, loin pain. These may indicate emboli caused by transfusion reaction.

Breathing

Pulse, respiration rates and blood pressure should be monitored, normally hourly, during the transfusion. Respiratory function should not be affected unless a transfusion reaction occurs or the blood is transfused at a rate which causes fluid overload (see Intravenous infusion, p.104).

Patients who have congestive cardiac failure should be transfused at an appropriately slower rate to prevent fluid overload with associated pulmonary oedema and dyspnoea; diuretics are sometimes prescribed during the transfusion to prevent this complication. The use of concentrated red cells instead of whole blood will help prevent fluid overload.

Eating and drinking

An accurate chart of fluid intake should be maintained.

The patient may need help with placing and preparing food if one hand is immobilised (see Intravenous infusion, p. 104).

Personal cleansing and dressing

Skin colour should be noted and abnormalities reported, e.g. pallor, flushing, rash, which may indicate transfusion reaction.

The patient may need some help with personal cleansing and dressing while one arm may be immobilised.

The need for light clothing allowing access to the transfusion site should be explained.

Relevance to the
activities of living
continued

Eliminating

Urine should be accurately measured to maintain fluid balance charts.

Diuresis may occur if diuretic medication is ordered; this should be explained.

If any incompatibility occurs the kidneys may be the first organs to be affected, because emboli may form in the renal capillaries due to clumping of incompatible blood. The patient may complain of back pain and there may be frank haematuria, which should be reported immediately.

The patient may need help, when using a commode, to support the administration tubing while the transfusion is in progress.

Controlling body temperature

Body temperature should be monitored hourly or as ordered; one of the early signs of adverse reaction may be a sudden rise in body temperature. Often this is associated with rigor, and either chilling or flushing is experienced by the patient.

Appropriate clothing and covering will help the patient to feel more comfortable.

Donor blood only remains stable at 1–6°C and should not be warmed prior to transfusion. In emergencies when a rapid transfusion is needed, special blood warming equipment is used, ordered by the medical practitioner. This is usually confined to transfusions occurring in accident and emergency units, the operating theatre, and intensive care areas.

In non-acute situations transfusions are normally prescribed at a flow rate of one unit every 4 hours. This slower rate of transfusion allows the body to adjust to the initially cold temperature of the donor blood.

Maintaining an accurate flow rate will help the patient to control body temperature.

Mobilising

Degree of mobility may depend on other factors. Initially it may be appropriate for the patient to rest comfortably, and this allows more accurate recordings and observations to be maintained.

The patient may move around the bed, sit in a chair and use a commode with help, as his condition allows.

Sleeping

Any change in the patient's general state of consciousness should be noted, e.g. confusion, restlessness, or disorientation, which may indicate transfusion reaction.

The patient may find it difficult to lie in his normal sleeping position, due to the transfusion lines. Help may be needed in adjusting to a suitable comfortable position.

Necessary observations may waken the patient. Temperature recordings may need to be maintained. A continuous recording with an electronic probe may be less disturbing than an intermittent recording with a mercury thermometer. The blood pressure may be recorded less frequently, during the sleeping period, as the patients' condition allows, if the pulse recording is continued, causing less disturbance.

Suggested reading

Chilman A, Thomas M 1987 Understanding nursing care, 3rd edn. Churchill Livingstone, Edinburgh, pp 316–319
Cluroe S 1989 Blood transfusion. Nursing 3(40) August: 8–11
Miller J A 1989 Transfusion of blood and blood products. Professional Nurse 4(11) August: 560, 562–565
Roper N, Logan W, Tierney A 1990 The elements of nursing, 3rd edn. Churchill Livingstone, Edinburgh, pp 136–142
Swaffield L 1987 Circulating the blood (Transfusion service and AIDS). Nursing Times 83(21) March 18: 16–17

Central Venous Pressure

There are two parts to this section:

1   Insertion of a central venous catheter
2   Measuring and recording central venous pressure

The concluding subsection 'Relevance to the activities of living', refers to both practices.

Objectives

By the end of this section you should know how to:

- prepare the patient for this nursing practice
- collect and prepare the equipment
- assist the medical practitioner with safe insertion of the central venous catheter
- measure, and record central venous pressure
- maintain the catheter in situ for a period of time

Related information

Revision of the anatomy and physiology of the cardiovascular system especially the heart, main vessels, and the veins of the neck and upper thorax.

Revision of intravenous therapy (see p. 104).

Revision of aseptic technique (see p. 26).

Review of health authority policy in relation to central venous pressure.

Some indications for monitoring central venous pressure

Central venous pressure (CVP) recording is the measurement of the pressure in the right atrium of the heart and is measured in cmH_2O. The pressure recorded reflects the circulatory fluid volume, and assessment of this may be required for seriously ill patients where close monitoring of fluid balance is needed. It may be indicated:

- for preoperative monitoring of patients who have haemorrhage or trauma
- for postoperative monitoring following major surgery, especially when intravenous therapy or parenteral nutrition are being administered
- for patients who have severe dehydration to monitor fluid replacement therapy, e.g. following vomiting, diarrhoea or haemorrhage
- for patients who have cardiogenic, bacteraemic or hypovolaemic shock
- for patients who have cardiac disease, to monitor fluid overload
- for patients who have renal disease, to monitor fluid overload
- for patients who have acute renal failure during haemodialysis or ultrafiltration procedures

1   INSERTION OF A CENTRAL VENOUS CATHETER

Outline of the procedure

This procedure is carried out by a medical practitioner using aseptic technique. The procedure involves the passage of a catheter through the veins to the superior vena cava, so that the tip of the catheter lies at the entrance of the right atrium of the heart (Fig. 3.14). The catheter is then connected to the manometer and giving set and an intravenous infusion is commenced (see Parenteral nutrition, p. 174).

Figure 3.14
Central venous pressure:
position of catheter in relation
to the heart

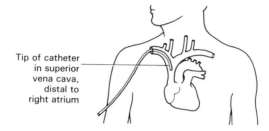

Tip of catheter
in superior
vena cava,
distal to
right atrium

The position of the patient

The position of the patient is important during this procedure, and is dependent on the choice of the entry site for catheterisation. There are three main entry sites (the first two are used more frequently):

The subclavian vein: The patient lies supine with his arms by his side. The head of the bed is lowered by 10°.

The internal jugular vein: The patient lies supine, with no pillow. The neck is extended. The head is rotated away from the site of entry, and well supported in position. The head of the bed is lowered by 10°. This position is important to prevent the danger of an air embolus occurring.

The median cephalic vein: The patient lies supine. The chosen arm is extended with the palm upwards and the elbow supported.

Ideally this procedure should be performed in theatre. If it is performed in the ward, it should take place in the treatment room.

Equipment

As for intravenous infusion (see p. 104).

Additional equipment

Theatre cap and mask
Sterile gown
Sterile gloves
Minor operation sterile pack or sterile drape and towels
Waterproof protection for the bed
Alcohol-based antiseptic for cleansing the skin
Venous pressure manometer set
Non-viscous sterile intravenous fluid, e.g. normal saline, dextrose 5% (this will be prescribed by the medical practitioner)
Appropriate sterile catheter depending on the site of entry used, e.g.:
A single, double or triple lumen catheter (Fig. 3.15)
Sterile needles and black silk sutures
ECG monitoring equipment if required
Local anaesthetic and equipment for its administration

Figure 3.15
Triple lumen catheter

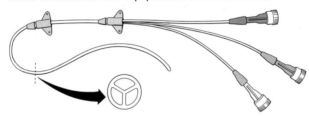

Guidelines for this nursing practice

Refer to the section on intravenous therapy (see p. 104) for detailed guidelines.

- help to explain the procedure to the patient and gain his consent and cooperation

- ensure the patient's privacy

- prepare the equipment and prime the administration set with the prescribed infusion fluid

- help the patient into the correct position depending on the site of entry used

- observe the patient throughout this activity

- adjust the angle of the bed, so that the patient's head is lowered if required

- protect the bed with waterproof material

- assist the medical practitioner as required

- remain with the patient and help to maintain his position

- commence the infusion of prescribed fluid once the catheter is in position and connected to the manometer and administration set. If a double or triple lumen catheter is used, the line designated for CVP recording is connected to the appropriate administration set and manometer, and labelled accordingly

- ensure the patient is left feeling as comfortable as possible

- dispose of the equipment safely

- document the procedure appropriately, monitor after-effects and report abnormal findings immediately

- maintain the infusion at the rate prescribed (see Intravenous infusion, p. 104)

A portable chest X-ray is taken as soon as possible after catheter insertion. A temporary sterile dressing may be applied until this has been performed. The catheter is usually held in place with skin sutures once it is judged to be correctly positioned, and a sterile transparent dressing applied over the site.

Occasionally arrhythmias may occur, due to irritation of the heart by the passage of the catheter, and observations may be supplemented by ECG monitoring. The rhythm usually returns to normal once the catheter is in the correct position.

2   MEASURING AND RECORDING CENTRAL VENOUS PRESSURE

The central venous pressure is measured in cmH_2O.

The range of normal is between 3–10 cmH_2O.

The central venous pressure (CVP) may be measured hourly, 2-hourly or 4-hourly depending on the patient's condition.

Equipment

A central venous catheter, intravenous fluid and associated lines in situ (Fig. 3.16)
A venous pressure manometer (Fig. 3.16)
A spirit level

Figure 3.16
Central venous pressure: position of the patient showing the catheter, manometer and 3-way stopcock when reading a central venous pressure

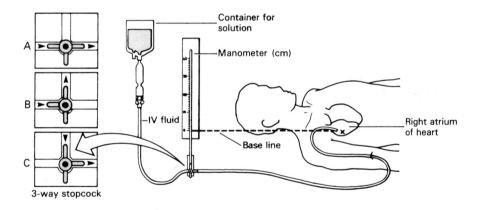

Guidelines for this nursing practice

- explain the nursing practice to the patient and gain his consent and cooperation

- ensure the patient's privacy

- help the patient into the correct position (Fig. 3.16). It is preferable for the patient to lie flat for absolute accuracy, as this position will prevent upward pressure of the abdominal organs affecting the reading. However, if lying flat causes the patient any distress an acceptable reading can be obtained with the patient sitting comfortably at an angle of about 45°. His body should be straight, with his shoulders flat against the back of the bed. The thorax must not be turned or twisted or a false reading may result

- position the manometer. It should be supported on a pole so that it is easily read, while still allowing the patient freedom of movement in bed between readings. There should be no strain on the lines or the catheter

- observe the patient throughout this activity

- assess the baseline. The level above which measurement of central venous pressure is taken is level with the patient's right atrium where the tip of the catheter is lying. The medical practitioner will note the level at an imaginary 90° angle between the sternal notch and the midline from the axilla. This can be marked on the patient's skin with his consent

- read the baseline. A spirit level is used to record the level on the manometer gauge which corresponds with the baseline level, which may be marked on the side of the patient's chest

- turn off all other infusions. Ideally only the CVP fluid should be infused through the CVP line, but on occasions other fluids are infused through the same line. The use of multiple lumen lines overcomes this problem. The tap of the three-way stopcock should be at position A between recordings and before commencing reading (Fig. 3.16)

Guidelines for this
nursing practice
continued

- flush the line to ensure patency and to clear all other infusions

- turn the tap on the three-way stopcock away from the patient, towards the infusion fluid to position B (Fig. 3.16); this allows the manometer tube to refill with fluid

- turn the tap towards the patient to position C (Fig. 3.16); this allows a free flow of fluid between the manometer tube and the catheter to be established. The fluid in the manometer tube will fall to a level which corresponds to the pressure in the right atrium or superior vena cava. The fluid fluctuates in relation to the patient's respirations once it falls to the level for recording

- read the level of the lower fluctuation on the manometer gauge once the fluid in the tube maintains a steady level with a fluctuation of 0.2–1.0 cm

- subtract the baseline reading from this figure; the resultant figure is the measurement of central venous pressure

- turn the tap on the stopcock back to position A (Fig. 3.16) to occlude the manometer and recommence the infusion fluid at the prescribed rate

- ensure that the patient is left feeling as comfortable as possible

- document the nursing practice appropriately, monitor after-effects and report abnormal findings immediately. A single reading is not as valuable as monitoring a series of recordings. These will show whether the central venous pressure is rising, falling or remaining steady

Pressure transducers

Increasingly, pressure transducers are being used to monitor the central venous pressure. The principles of the practice, the care of the patient, and the care of the lines are exactly the same. The pressure transducer and the appropriate lines are substituted for the manometer set. The measurement is recorded on a bedside monitor screen. When a reading is taken the height of the transducer, which is supported on a pole, is adjusted to be level with the assessed baseline, as previously described.

Central Venous Pressure

Relevance to the activities of living

As for intravenous infusion and in addition:

Maintaining a safe environment

A central venous catheter gives direct access to the heart so the dangers from infection are increased. Meticulous care for the prevention of infection must be maintained at all times. Aseptic technique should be used whenever dressings, infusions or lines are changed. Good hand washing technique should be used before touching the equipment for measuring the central venous pressure.

The nurse should ensure that the lines do not become disconnected, otherwise air may enter and create an air embolus. The lines should be observed for air bubbles and appropriate action taken. The danger from an air embolus is increased because of the direct access to the heart.

The nurse should ensure that the line remains patent, and the infusion is maintained at the required rate to help prevent clotting or occlusion of the line (see Intravenous therapy, p. 104).

Breathing

The central venous pressure is at the lower level of normal in young healthy adults. It increases slightly with age.

It is raised in patients who have respiratory disease, due to the increased intrapulmonary pressure.

It is significantly raised in patients with bronchospasm, e.g. asthma, as this increases the intrathoracic pressure and may mask any change in circulatory fluid volume.

It is raised in patients with congestive cardiac failure due to the increase in circulatory fluid volume.

A rare complication would be the development of a pneumothorax. This is more likely to occur at the time of insertion of the catheter. Any sudden change in the patient's general condition or respiratory function should be reported immediately.

Eating and drinking

The central venous pressure reflects the volume of circulating fluid and any fluid imbalance; it is lowered in patients who are dehydrated and raised in patients with fluid overload. Accurate recordings of fluid intake should be maintained during the period of monitoring central venous pressure.

Eliminating

Accurate recordings of fluid output should be maintained during the period of monitoring, for assessment of the patient's fluid balance.

The central venous pressure is raised in patients who have renal disease; it will show a temporary fall during a period of treatment with diuretic medication.

Personal cleansing and dressing

While attached to the manometer the patient may need appropriate help with personal cleansing. The necessity for wearing light clothing which allows unrestricted access to the site of catheterisation should be explained to the patient.

Controlling body temperature

The dangers of infection are increased during this procedure, as the central line has direct access to the heart. The patient's temperature should be recorded 2-hourly or 4-hourly during the period of CVP monitoring, to observe any signs of developing infection. This should continue to be monitored 4-hourly for 48 hours after the central line has been removed.

Mobilising

The central venous pressure will not be affected by the patient moving around the bed between readings. He may be helped into a chair with the manometer and lines adequately supported, as his condition allows.

Suggested reading

Davidson L 1986 Dressing subclavian catheters. Nursing Times 82(7) February 12: 40
Darbyshire P 1988 Making sense of ... central venous catheters. Nursing Times 84(6) 36–38
Goodison S 1990 Keeping the flora out. Professional Nurse 5(11) August: 572–575
Pike S 1989 Family participation in the care of central lines. Nursing 3(38) June: 22–25
Roper N, Logan W, Tierney A 1990 The elements of nursing, 3rd edn. Churchill Livingstone, Edinburgh, pp 136–142
Speer E W 1990 Central venous catheterisation. Issues associated with the use of single and multilumen catheters. Journal of Intravenous Nursing 13(1) January/February: 30–39

Chest Aspiration

Objectives

By the end of this section you should know how to:

- prepare the patient for this nursing practice
- collect and prepare the equipment
- assist the medical practitioner during chest aspiration

Related information

Revision of the anatomy and physiology of the respiratory system.

Revision of aseptic technique (see p. 26).

Some indications for aspirating the pleural cavity

The lungs are covered by the visceral pleura and the inner chest wall is lined by the parietal pleura. Between these pleura is a thin layer of serous fluid whose surface tension holds the two pleural linings together. As a result, the lung follows the movement of the chest wall and lung volume is determined by the size of the thorax. An increase of fluid in the space upsets this mechanism. Chest aspiration involves the introduction of a needle into the pleural cavity between the visceral and parietal pleura. It may be performed for the following reasons:

- to examine a specimen of the pleural fluid as an aid to the diagnosis of disease, e.g. tuberculosis, carcinoma
- to relieve dyspnoea, by removing excess pleural fluid
- to introduce medication into the pleural cavity, e.g. antibiotics

Outline of the procedure

Using aseptic technique, the medical practitioner washes and dries his hands, cleanses the patient's skin over the selected site of entry of the aspiration needle, injects a local anaesthetic and waits for it to take effect. He then inserts the aspiration needle into the cavity between the visceral and parietal layers of the pleura (Fig. 3.17). After withdrawing the stilette from the needle, specimens of fluid can be obtained from the cavity for laboratory investigation, and the remaining fluid may be allowed to drain out. If the fluid is purulent, it may have to be aspirated by attaching a large syringe to the needle. At the end of the procedure the aspirating needle is withdrawn, a sterile plastic spray applied to the wound puncture, and an adhesive dressing applied.

Figure 3.17
Aspiration of pleural fluid (Reproduced with permission from Chilman A, Thomas M (eds) 1987 Understanding nursing care, 3rd edn. Churchill Livingstone, Edinburgh)

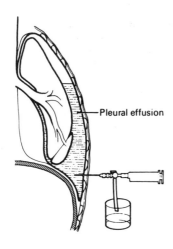

Pleural effusion

Equipment

Trolley
Sterile dressings pack
Sterile gloves
Alcohol-based antiseptic for skin cleansing
Local anaesthetic, and equipment for its administration
50 ml sterile syringe
Sterile aspiration needles
Sterile two-way tap with length of sterile rubber tubing
Sterile bowl for collecting fluid
Sterile specimen bottles, appropriately labelled
Laboratory form
Plastic specimen bag for transportation
Sterile plastic spray and adhesive dressing
Receptacle for soiled disposables

Chest Aspiration

Guidelines for this nursing practice

- help to explain the procedure to the patient and obtain his consent and cooperation
- ensure the patient's privacy
- collect the equipment
- administer a sedative if prescribed by medical staff
- help the patient into a back-fastening gown
- assist the patient to sit up with his arms extended over a bed table on which a pillow has been placed for him to rest his head. If this is not comfortable for the patient he may be encouraged to lie in bed on the unaffected side
- observe the patient throughout this activity
- open the sterile equipment as it is required by medical staff
- remain with the patient and help him maintain his position as required
- observe the patient's respirations and any complaints of pain during the procedure
- ensure the patient is left feeling as comfortable as possible
- dispose of equipment safely
- dispatch the labelled specimen container in a plastic specimen bag immediately to the laboratory with the completed form
- document this nursing practice appropriately, monitor after-effects and report abnormal findings immediately

Relevance to the activities of living

Maintaining a safe environment

This is an invasive procedure and all precautions for the prevention of infection must be taken. A meticulous technique should be used and thorough hand washing should be carried out, preferably using an antiseptic detergent. For the safe transport of specimens see Specimen collection, p. 198.

During and after this procedure there is some risk of a pneumothorax occurring, so the patient should be observed closely and a chest X-ray performed. A pneumothorax is a collapse of the lung due to atmospheric air entering the pleural space and causing the loss of the normally negative intrathoracic pressure. The clinical features are chest pain, rapid respirations, and dyspnoea.

Breathing

By removing excess fluid from the pleural cavity and allowing the lungs to expand during inspiration, this procedure should help to relieve some of the patient's breathing problems and alleviate attendant pain.

Controlling body temperature

If infection is present in the pleural space the patient may have an elevated temperature. Tepid sponging may help to reduce the temperature to within normal range (see p. 286 for tepid sponging).

Mobilising

The chest aspiration as such would not alter the patient's ability to mobilise but he is usually advised to rest for 4–6 hours following the procedure.

Suggested reading   Duthie J 1984 Anatomy and physiology of respiration. Nursing 2(27) July: 785–787
Hamilton H (ed) 1985 Nurse's reference library – procedures. Springhouse
    Corporation, Pennsylvania, pp 500–502

Underwater Seal Chest Drainage

There are three parts to this section:

1 **Insertion of an underwater seal chest drain**
2 **Changing a chest drainage bottle**
3 **Removal of an underwater seal chest drain**

The concluding subsection, 'Relevance to the activities of living', refers to the three practices collectively.

Objectives

By the end of this section you should know how to:

- prepare the patient for these three nursing practices

- collect and prepare the equipment necessary to insert a chest drain and connect it to underwater seal drainage; change a chest drainage bottle; and remove an underwater seal chest drain

- assist the medical practitioner in parts 1 and 3

- care for the patient who has a chest drain connected to underwater seal drainage

Related information

Revision of the anatomy and physiology of the respiratory system.

Revision of aseptic technique (see p. 26).

1   INSERTION OF AN UNDERWATER SEAL CHEST DRAIN

Underwater seal chest drainage is a closed system of drainage which allows air or fluid to pass in one direction only, i.e. from the pleural space to the collecting bottle. It may be established in the following circumstances:

- to bring about re-expansion of the lung when there is air or fluid, e.g. blood or pus, in the pleural space as a result of injury, surgery or a respiratory disease or dysfunction

Outline of the procedure

Using an aseptic technique, the medical practitioner washes and dries his hands, cleanses the patient's skin over the selected site of entry for the drain, injects a local anaesthetic and waits for it to take effect. He then makes a small incision with the scalpel, inserts the drain and introducer, removes the introducer and connects the drain to the equipment already prepared by the nurse. A purse-string suture is inserted round the entry site of the drain to seal off the site when the drain is eventually removed. A dressing is usually placed over the site to help prevent infection of the small wound (Fig. 3.18).

If there is air in the pleural space, the drain is usually inserted at the level of the 3rd or 4th intercostal space. The insertion site is lower if fluid has gathered in the pleural space, to promote maximum drainage.

Figure 3.18
Underwater seal chest drainage
A Drainage system in position
B Detail of the position of the catheter

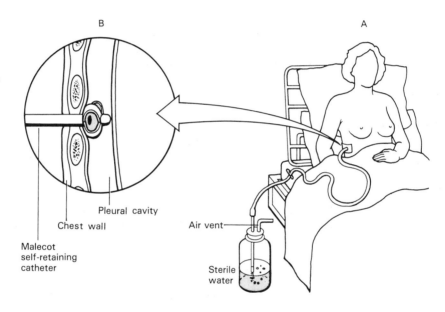

B   A

Pleural cavity

Chest wall   Air vent

Malecot
self-retaining
catheter

Sterile
water

Equipment

Trolley
Sterile dressings pack
Alcohol-based antiseptic for skin cleansing
Local anaesthetic and equipment for administration
Sterile scalpel and blade
Sterile black silk suture
Sterile chest drain and introducer
Sterile drainage bottle, cap, glass or plastic rods and tubing
500 ml sterile water or normal saline
2 pairs tubing clamps
Receptacle for soiled disposables

Guidelines for this nursing practice

- help to explain the procedure to the patient and gain his consent and cooperation
- ensure the patient's privacy
- administer a sedative if prescribed by medical staff
- collect the equipment
- help the patient into the position suggested by the medical staff
- observe the patient throughout this activity
- put sterile water into the chest drainage bottle and fasten the cap with long and short rods inserted and tubing connected to the long rod, the end of which should be below water level. The tubing should be clamped until all the equipment is connected. Ensure that the tubing is long enough to allow free movement
- open the sterile equipment and help the medical practitioner as requested
- seal all connections with waterproof tape, if required, to ensure that they are airtight

- ensure that the collection bottle is always below the level of the patient's chest so that there is no reflux into the pleural space (Fig. 3.19)
- release the clamps when connected to the drain and satisfied that there are no air leaks at the connections
- check that the apparatus is functioning; the fluid should be oscillating in the long under-water tube in time with the patient's respirations. If positive suction is required, connect a second drainage bottle by tubing from its long rod to the short rod of the first. The short rod of the second drainage bottle is then connected by tubing to a suction machine, the pressure of which has been decided by the medical practitioner (Fig. 3.19)
- apply a sterile dressing to the wound site
- ensure the patient is left feeling as comfortable as possible
- dispose of the equipment safely
- document the procedure appropriately, monitor after-effects and report abnormal findings immediately

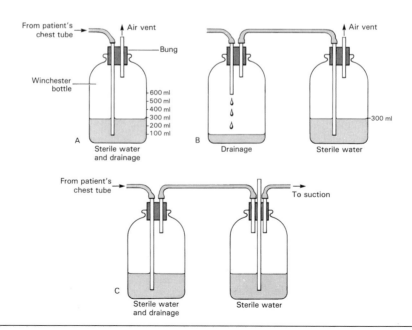

Figure 3.19
Underwater seal chest drainage system
A Using one bottle
B Using two bottles
C Using two bottles plus suction

2   CHANGING A CHEST DRAINAGE BOTTLE

Some indications for changing a drainage bottle

As drainage from the pleural space accumulates and approaches the three-quarters full level, the drainage bottle has to be changed:

- to enable the equipment to continue functioning efficiently

Equipment

Sterile drainage bottle, cap, glass or plastic rods and tubing
500 ml sterile water or normal saline
Receptacle for soiled disposables

Guidelines for this nursing practice

- collect and prepare the equipment
- explain this practice to the patient
- observe the patient throughout this activity
- clamp off the intercostal drain securely with the two pairs of clamps
- disconnect the tubing
- connect fresh tubing and apparatus
- ensure that all connections are airtight and that the drainage bottle is below chest level

- release the clamps and check the oscillation of fluid in the underwater tube
- ensure the patient is left feeling as comfortable as possible
- dispose of the equipment safely
- document this nursing practice appropriately, monitor effects, and report abnormal findings immediately

3 REMOVAL OF AN UNDERWATER SEAL CHEST DRAIN

Some indications for removal of an underwater seal chest drain

Underwater seal drainage is a temporary measure and is removed:

- when radiological examination demonstrates that the patient's lung has fully re-inflated

Equipment

Trolley
Sterile dressings pack
Sterile stitch cutter
Water-based antiseptic for wound cleansing
Waterproof tape and scissors
Sterile artery forceps
Receptacle for soiled disposables

Guidelines for this nursing practice

Two nurses, one of whom must be qualified, or the nurse and a medical practitioner are required to carry out this practice.

- explain the nursing practice to the patient and gain his consent and cooperation

- ensure the patient's privacy

- administer a sedative if it is prescribed by the medical practitioner

- collect the equipment

- prepare and assist the patient into a suitable position which is as comfortable as possible

- observe the patient throughout this activity

- remove the dressing from the drain site

- clean the drain site with the antiseptic

- clamp the ends of the purse-string suture with the artery forceps to facilitate tightening the suture

- raise the drain slightly (performed by the assistant) while the qualified practitioner cuts and removes the retaining suture

- request the patient to breathe in and while he is breathing out the qualified practitioner holds folded swabs over the puncture site with one hand and with the dominant hand pulls the drain out quickly and smoothly. The assistant tightens the purse string suture as the drain is removed

- remove the artery forceps from the end of the purse string suture and knot it

- apply a sterile dressing and waterproof tape

- order a chest X-ray to ensure that the lung is functioning normally

- ensure the patient is left feeling as comfortable as possible

- dispose of the equipment safely

- document the nursing practice, monitor after-effects and report abnormal findings immediately

**Relevance to the
activities of living**

Maintaining a safe environment

A meticulous technique must be used for the prevention of infection. Thorough handwashing should be carried out, preferably using an antiseptic detergent.

Ensure that the tubing is not being compressed or kinked by the patient lying on it, as this will cause the equipment to function inefficiently.

It is imperative that the drainage bottle is kept below the level of the patient's chest, unless double clamped, or there may be a back flow of fluid into the pleural cavity.

When the drain is being removed, care must be taken to prevent a pneumothorax occurring (i.e. the entry of air into the pleural space).

Communicating

Because of breathlessness, the patient may have difficulty in talking. A pencil and paper may help him to communicate with staff, and a bell should always be to hand to summon assistance if necessary. Analgesia may be prescribed to help relieve any pain or discomfort.

Breathing

If the equipment is functioning correctly, after the insertion of the drain, the patient's respiratory rate should gradually return to his normal range.

The patient's respirations should be closely monitored after removal of the drain so that the potential complication of pneumothorax can be detected quickly.

Personal cleansing and dressing

Some assistance with washing and dressing may have to be given to patients who are attached to underwater seal drainage equipment as their mobility is reduced. Light loose clothing should be worn so that breathing is not unduly impaired.

Mobilising

Movement will be restricted by the equipment but the patient should be encouraged to be as independent as possible.

Sleeping

The patient's normal sleeping pattern may be altered because of difficulty with breathing and because of the presence of the equipment, so the nurse should take measures which help to induce sleep.

Suggested reading

Allan D 1985 Chest tube patients. Nursing Times 85(24) June 14: 40–41
Brunner L, Suddarth D 1986 The Lippincott manual of nursing practices. J.B. Lippincott, Philadelphia, pp 181–184
Hamilton H (ed) 1985 Nurse's reference library – procedures. Springhouse Corporation, Pennsylvania, pp 502–510
Nicoll J 1983 Management of underwater seal chest drainage. Nursing Times February 23: 58–59
Walsh M 1989 Making Sense of chest drainage. Nursing Times 85(24) June 14: 40–41

Tracheostomy Care

There are two parts to this section:

1 Removal of respiratory tract secretions via a tracheostomy tube
2 Changing a tracheostomy tube

The concluding subsection, 'Relevance to the activities of living', refers to both practices.

Objectives

By the end of this section you should know how to:

- prepare the patient for this nursing practice
- collect and prepare the equipment
- care for a patient who has a tracheostomy tube in situ

Related information

Revision of the anatomy and physiology of the larynx, trachea, bronchus.

Revision of aseptic technique (see p. 26).

Review of health authority policy on care of a patient with a tracheostomy.

Some indications for tracheostomy care

Tracheostomy describes the surgical procedure of creating an artificial opening into the trachea to relieve an obstruction of the airway (e.g. tumour, acute infection). This procedure is almost always performed in an operating theatre. The artificial airway is maintained with a suitable tube and this requires to be aspirated, cleaned and changed:

- to ensure the tube remains patent
- to reduce the risk of respiratory infection

1 REMOVAL OF RESPIRATORY TRACT SECRETIONS VIA A TRACHEOSTOMY TUBE

Equipment

Tray
Sterile disposable gloves
Sterile suction catheters with a thumb control
Sterile container and water for flushing the catheter and tubing
Receptacle for soiled disposables
Suction apparatus, e.g. portable machine or wall suction

Guidelines for this nursing practice

- explain the nursing practice to the patient, if possible, and gain his consent and cooperation

- ensure the patient's privacy

- collect the equipment

- assist the patient to a suitable position

- observe the patient throughout this activity

- fill the sterile container with sterile water

- open the end of the pack containing the suction catheter and connect it to the tubing of the suction machine

- put a disposable glove on the dominant hand

- slide the cover off the catheter and rinse it through with sterile water to lubricate it

- insert the catheter into the tracheostomy for 20–25 cm with the gloved hand and without any suction (Fig. 3.20)

- withdraw the catheter, applying suction by covering the thumb control hole and rotate the catheter as this is being done. If the mucus is tenacious and difficult to remove, medical staff may order 5–15 ml of sterile normal saline to be dripped into the tracheostomy before suction is applied

- allow the patient to rest and re-oxygenate before repeating insertion of the catheter

- dispose of the catheter at the end of the practice after rinsing it and the tubing with sterile water

- ensure that the patient is left feeling as comfortable as possible

- dispose of the equipment safely

- document the nursing practice appropriately, monitor after-effects, and report abnormal findings immediately

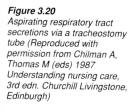

Figure 3.20
Aspirating respiratory tract secretions via a tracheostomy tube (Reproduced with permission from Chilman A, Thomas M (eds) 1987 Understanding nursing care, 3rd edn. Churchill Livingstone, Edinburgh)

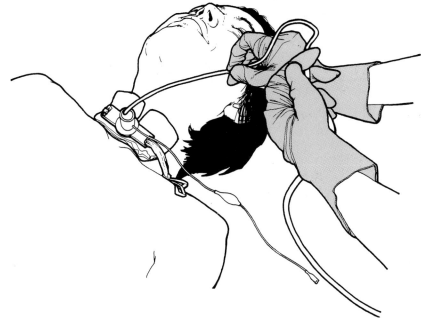

2   CHANGING A TRACHEOSTOMY TUBE

Equipment

Tray or trolley
Sterile dressings pack
2 sterile tracheostomy tubes, taped and with an obturator
Sterile KY jelly
Sterile tracheal dilators
Sterile scissors
Protective pad
Container of sodium bicarbonate solution in which to put the soiled silver tracheostomy tube
Disposable gloves
Instrument brush
Receptacle for soiled disposables

Plastic disposable tracheostomy tubes are normally used nowadays for temporary tracheostomies. Silver tubes are still preferred by most surgeons and patients for use in permanent tracheostomies because the wide range of sizes and types makes it possible to choose the one most suitable for each patient (Fig. 3.21).

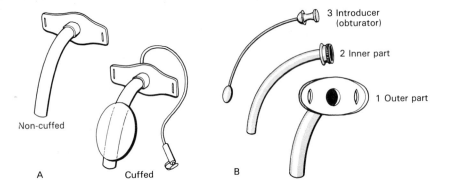

Figure 3.21
Tracheostomy tubes in common use
A Disposable
B Non-disposable

Non-cuffed

A   Cuffed   B

3 Introducer (obturator)
2 Inner part
1 Outer part

Guidelines for this nursing practice

- explain the nursing practice to the patient and gain his consent and cooperation
- ensure the patient's privacy
- collect and prepare the equipment
- assist the patient to a suitable position
- observe the patient throughout this activity
- open the dressings pack and the tracheostomy tube pack
- check that the obturator fits
- lubricate the end of the tube and obturator
- make a slit in the end of the protective pad
- put on the disposable gloves
- remove the soiled tube with a smooth outward and downward motion, discarding it into the receptacle for disposables if it is plastic, *or* putting it into a container of sodium bicarbonate solution if it is silver

- remove the gloves
- hold the new tube by the tapes and insert it smoothly from below in an upwards, in and down movement into the trachea
- immediately remove the obturator while holding the tube in place
- tie the tapes at the side of the patient's neck
- slide the protective pad into position round the stoma
- ensure that the patient is left feeling as comfortable as possible
- dispose of the equipment safely
- clean the soiled tube using the brush and gloved hands if a silver tube is used
- record this nursing practice appropriately, monitor after-effects, and report abnormal findings immediately

Tracheostomy Care

Relevance to the activities of living

Maintaining a safe environment

All precautions must be taken for the prevention of infection, as the air inhaled via the tracheostomy tube bypasses the protective ciliated epithelium of the nose, and so increases the risk of pulmonary infection. The wound must also be protected from sources of infection.

Thorough hand washing should be carried out, preferably using an antiseptic detergent.

The suction catheter must be inserted gently, and the prescribed suction pressure must not be exceeded or the tracheal mucosa may be traumatised.

Tracheal dilators should be available when changing the tube of a patient with a newly-formed tracheostomy, in case there is difficulty inserting the new tube. This is a rare occurrence.

Care must be taken to maintain a clear airway at all times, as the tube interferes with the normal cough reflex. The need for suctioning may be detected visually (the appearance of laboured breathing, increase in rate, change in pattern), aurally (moist, gurgling sounds) or by auscultation (low-pitched, loose rattling).

Communicating

A tracheostomy reduces the function of the vocal cords, so the patient may have a problem with verbal communication, but the use of a pad of paper and pencil may partially overcome this. A bell must always be available for the patient to summon assistance.

If it is envisaged that the tracheostomy will be permanent, a teaching programme to educate the patient to change his own tube may be planned and implemented, by suitably qualified staff.

Breathing

The purpose of a tracheostomy is to aid the patient's breathing, but the nurse must be vigilant to ensure the patency of the tube at all times.

If a silver tracheostomy tube is used, it will have an inner lining. It may be sufficient to remove this on alternate days and clean it thoroughly with sodium bicarbonate solution, sterilise and re-insert it after applying suction to clear the outer tube.

Eating and drinking

As the trachea is in close proximity, anatomically, to the upper alimentary organs, the presence of a tracheostomy tube may cause apprehension about swallowing, and education and encouragement should be given to the patient to maintain dietary intake.

Personal cleansing and dressing

Advice may be required about the most suitable type of clothing to wear around the stoma and about skin care of the stoma area especially if the tracheostomy is permanent. The tapes should be tied at the side of the neck, not over the cervical spine where the knot causes discomfort.

Expressing sexuality

A permanent tracheostomy may cause the patient to have psychological problems due to altered body image. A talk with someone who has successfully adjusted to life with a tracheostomy can help.

Sleeping

Initially the patient may be unwilling to sleep, fearing that the tube may become blocked, and reassurance that staff are available and observing may have to be given to relieve such anxiety.

Suggested reading

Allan D 1987 Making sense of tracheostomy. Nursing Times 83(45) November 11: 36–38

De Carle B 1985 Tracheostomy care. Nursing Times 81(40) October 2: 50–54

Gibson I 1983 Tracheostomy management. Nursing 2 (18) October: 538–540

Harris R, Hyman R 1984 Clean *v.* sterile tracheostomy care and level of pulmonary infection. Nursing Research 33(2) March/April: 80

Roper N, Logan W, Tierney A 1990 The elements of nursing, 3rd edn. Churchill Livingstone, Edinburgh, pp 151–152

Sorensen K, Luckmann J 1986 Basic nursing: a psychophysiologic approach. W. B. Saunders, Philadelphia, pp 920–930

Bone Marrow Aspiration

Objectives

By the end of this section you should know how to:

- prepare the patient for this procedure
- collect and prepare the equipment
- assist the medical practitioner during bone marrow aspiration

Related information

Revision of the anatomy and physiology of the blood with special reference to the source and development of the red blood corpuscles.

Revision of aseptic technique (see p. 26).

Some indications for bone marrow aspiration

Bone marrow aspiration is the aspiration of a specimen of red bone marrow:

- to aid diagnosis in some anaemias and leukaemias
- to aid assessment of the effect of treatment during the course of a disease

Outline of the procedure

This procedure is carried out by a medical practitioner using aseptic technique. The patient may have some form of sedation prescribed prior to the procedure. After washing his hands the medical practitioner administers the local anaesthetic into the chosen site. He then prepares his hands for the application of the sterile gloves. The patient's skin is cleansed using the antiseptic, a small stab incision may be made and the marrow needle is inserted into the red bone marrow cavity. The needle is specially designed and is fitted with an adjustable protective guard to control the level of penetration by the needle thus preventing injury to underlying vital organs (Fig. 3.22). The stilette of the needle is removed and the syringe attached to the hub of the marrow needle. Following aspiration of a specimen of red bone marrow, the syringe is disconnected, the stilette is replaced and the needle withdrawn. The microscope slides are prepared by the medical practitioner or a haematology technician if present. As the microscope slides are prepared, pressure should be applied to the puncture site until bleeding ceases. The puncture site may be sprayed with a plastic spray dressing prior to the application of an adhesive dressing.

The position of the patient during the procedure is dependent on the chosen site for aspiration of the red marrow. The main sites are:

The sternum: The patient lies supine with one pillow at his head.

The iliac crest: This can be either an anterior or posterior approach. If the anterior approach is used the patient can lie prone or on his side. When the posterior approach is used the patient must lie on his side. The iliac crest has the advantage of having no vital organs near the puncture site.

Figure 3.22
Bone marrow aspiration needle (disposable) showing adjustable guard
A Complete needle
B Needle taken apart

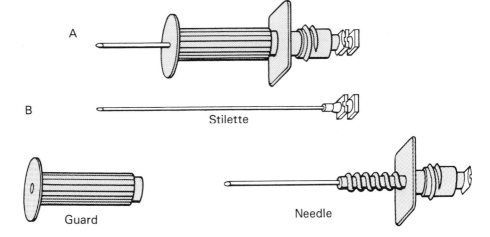

A

B   Stilette

Guard   Needle

Bone Marrow Aspiration

Equipment

Sterile gloves

Sterile dressings pack

Alcohol-based antiseptic for cleansing the skin

Local anaesthetic and equipment for its administration

Sterile disposable scalpel or similar equipment

Sterile marrow aspiration needles

Sterile 20 ml syringe for aspiration of the marrow

Plastic spray dressing

Sterile adhesive dressing

Trolley for equipment

Receptacle for soiled disposables

Microscope slides, appropriately labelled, coverslips and slide fixative if haematology technician service not available

Sterile specimen containers appropriately labelled with a completed laboratory form and plastic specimen bag for transportation

Guidelines for this nursing practice

- help to explain the procedure to the patient and gain his consent and cooperation

- wash the hands

- give the patient sedation if prescribed

- prepare the equipment and trolley as required

- ensure the patient's privacy

- help the patient into the correct position depending on the chosen site

- observe the patient throughout this activity

- assist the medical practitioner as necessary during the procedure

- remain with the patient and help maintain his position as required during the procedure

- ensure that the patient is left feeling as comfortable as possible

- dispose of the equipment safely

- dispatch the labelled specimens to the laboratory immediately with the completed laboratory forms

- document the nursing practice appropriately, monitor after-effects, and report abnormal findings immediately

Relevance to the activities of living

Maintaining a safe environment

As this is an invasive procedure all precautions and observations to prevent infection should be maintained. Unless a complication has arisen the adhesive dressing can be removed 2–3 days following the procedure.

For safe transportation of the specimen collected, see p. 198.

If the patient received sedation prior to the procedure, the effects of this should have worn off before he is allowed to mobilise.

Communicating

It is important that an easily understood explanation is given to the patient prior to the procedure. This is primarily given by the medical practitioner, but the nurse may be required to repeat the explanation. If the sternal site is used the thought of a needle being introduced into one's chest can be extremely alarming and if the patient is very anxious, the doctor may prescribe some light sedation prior to the procedure.

The patient should be told to expect a momentary sharp pain during the procedure when the syringe piston is withdrawn.

The patient may require mild analgesia once the effect of the local anaesthetic has worn off.

Breathing

The patient's blood pressure, pulse and respiration rates may be taken following bone marrow aspiration. The puncture site should be observed for continued bleeding or haematoma formation as some patients may have a bleeding disorder.

Any sudden change in the patient's general condition, especially in breathing if the sternal site is used, should be reported as this may signify injury to underlying vital organs.

Mobilising

The patient should be allowed to rest quietly for approximately an hour following the practice. Thereafter he can resume his previous form of mobilising. If sedation is given prior to the practice, allow the effects to wear off before the patient is mobilised.

Suggested reading

Booth J 1983 Handbook of investigations. Harper & Row, London, pp 49–51
Brunner L, Suddarth D 1988 Textbook of medical–surgical nursing, 6th edn. J. B. Lippincott Company, Philadelphia, pp 668–670
Chilman A, Thomas M 1981 Understanding nursing care, 3rd edn. Churchill Livingstone, Edinburgh, p 301
Faulkner A 1985 Nursing – a creative approach. Baillière Tindall, Eastbourne, p 162
Knowle S, Hoffbrand A 1980 Bone marrow aspiration and trephine biopsy. British Medical Journal 281(6234) July 19: 204–205
Roper N, Logan W, Tierney A 1990 The elements of nursing, 3rd edn. Churchill Livingstone, Edinburgh, ch 8

Cardiopulmonary Resuscitation

Objectives

By the end of this section you should know how to:

- diagnose cardiac arrest quickly
- call the emergency team promptly
- initiate resuscitation effectively
- locate the necessary equipment

Related information

Revision of the anatomy and physiology of the cardiovascular and respiratory systems.

Review of the health authority policy pertaining to the procedure of cardiopulmonary resuscitation.

Some indications for cardiopulmonary resuscitation

Cardiopulmonary resuscitation is a dramatic, emergency exercise to restore effective circulation and ventilation following cardiac arrest. Of the three levels of skill detailed under the AL of communicating the second is the level of knowledge expected of a nurse.

Cardiac arrest is the abrupt cessation of cardiac function, which may be induced by any of the following:

- respiratory failure as the cardiovascular and respiratory systems are so interdependent
- cardiac arrhythmias caused by cardiac disease or electrolyte imbalance
- surgery
- asphyxia
- accidents such as drowning or electrocution

Diagnosis of cardiac arrest is confirmed by:

- sudden loss of consciousness
- absence of the carotid pulse
- absence of respirations
- pallor often associated with cyanosis
- dilation of the pupils
- convulsions, which may or may not be present

Immediate cardiopulmonary resuscitation consists of three procedures. The mnemonic 'ABC' acts as an aide memoire:

A – Airway:
- providing and maintaining a clear airway

B – Breathing:
- supplying oxygen to the blood by means of artificial ventilation

C – Circulation:
- forcing the blood out of the heart into the arterial system by means of chest compression

Equipment

Suction equipment
Oral pharyngeal airway, e.g. Brook airway, Guedel airway
Ambubag and face mask or similar equipment
Oxygen equipment
Emergency cardiac medications
Defibrillator
Receptacle for soiled disposables

Guidelines for this nursing practice

- note the time, once cardiac arrest has been diagnosed
- order someone to alert the hospital cardiac arrest team and bring emergency equipment
- position the patient in a supine position on a firm surface
- remove the bedhead from the patient's bed

Support for breathing and circulation must be carried out simultaneously to be effective.

A = airway

- clear the airway using suction if required. Dentures to remain in situ if well fitting
- tilt the head backwards and pull the mandible forward to open the airway. Maintain this position (Fig. 3.23). If an injury to the cervical spine is suspected open the airway using the jaw thrust technique
- insert an oral airway

B = breathing

- two initial ventilations at 1–1.5 seconds per breath should be administered using the airway and Ambubag and/or bag mask
- note the rising of the chest wall to confirm ventilation
- ventilate at a rate of at least 12 per minute

Figure 3.23
Cardiopulmonary resuscitation
A Two resuscitators
B One resuscitator

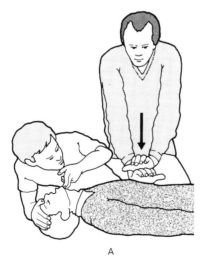
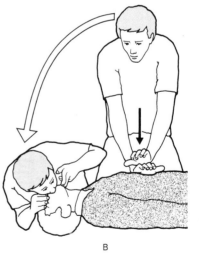

A

B

Guidelines for this
nursing practice
continued

C = circulation

- if the cardiac arrest is witnessed give one sharp blow over the mid-sternal area. This may cause the heart to restart

- check the carotid pulse; if absent continue

- place the heel of one hand over the lower half of the sternum

- place the other hand on top

- keeping the arms straight and elbows locked, depress the sternum 4–5 cm toward the spine (Fig. 3.23)

- repeat this movement at a rate of one depression per second

- continue chest compression and artificial ventilation at the rate of five chest compressions to one lung inflation when two nurses are resuscitating a patient. If only one person is carrying out the practice the ratio is 15:2, with a faster chest compression of 80 per minute because of the breaks for lung ventilation

- check for the return of the pulse and breathing after one minute and thereafter every three minutes

With the arrival of the cardiac arrest team the role of the nurses may alter. Breathing support is usually taken over by a medical practitioner, but chest compression is not always taken over. Nursing staff may thereafter:

- assist a medical practitioner with the passage of an endotracheal tube through which ventilation is continued

- assist a second medical practitioner with the commencement of an intravenous infusion to aid correction of the acid–base balance in the body and provide a route for administration of emergency medications

- assist if required with the application of limb or chest electrodes to provide continuous monitoring of cardiac function

- assist the medical practitioner to draw up emergency cardiac medications as required. A brief record of all medications administered should be kept. A defibrillator may be used by a medical practitioner during

cardiopulmonary resuscitation to help establish cardiac function or correct a cardiac arrhythmia. The defibrillator transmits an electric current through the patient's chest wall. All personnel must stand clear of the bed while the patient is being defibrillated because they may act as a 'ground' for the electric current, cancelling its usefulness and endangering the lives of the staff present

- ensure the patient is left feeling as comfortable as possible following successful resuscitation

- dispose of equipment safely

- document the nursing practice appropriately, monitor after-effects and report abnormal findings immediately

Relevance to the activities of living

Maintaining a safe environment

The brain tissue is most sensitive to the lack of blood and oxygen; and if an adequate cerebral circulation is not restored within three minutes, irreversible brain damage will occur. A nurse, when commencing work in a new ward, should primarily familiarise herself with the position of the equipment used in that ward during cardiopulmonary resuscitation.

Following cardiopulmonary resuscitation procedures, and at regular intervals, e.g. weekly, the equipment should be checked to ensure that it is in working condition and that stocks are replenished.

Communicating

It is now accepted that three levels of skill in cardiopulmonary resuscitation should be taught. The first is 'basic life support' which the population as a whole should learn. No equipment is necessary as the victim's airway is maintained and breathing and circulation supported by simple skills which can be easily taught.

The second level is 'basic life support with adjuncts' which all nurses should learn. The basic principles of life support are utilised with the additional use of an airway, Ambubag and mask. Nursing personnel working in high patient dependent units should also be taught the skills required for the use of a defibrillator.

The third level is 'advanced life support' which all cardiopulmonary resuscitation teams should be competent in delivering. This involves the implementation of internationally recognised recommendations for treatment regimens of the cause of a cardiac arrest.

Other patients witnessing any part of cardiopulmonary resuscitation will be alarmed and distressed. During the procedure, nurses who are not involved can give comfort and reassurance to these patients and wherever possible, continue with the normal work pattern.

Following this emergency the patient's next of kin should be contacted and informed.

When resuscitative measures are successful the patient will require a brief, easily understood explanation as to what has happened, and the reasons for the equipment which is being used.

Following such a dramatic emergency procedure, junior nursing staff may be distressed, and can be helped by supportive colleagues.

Breathing

A relatively common complication of external cardiac massage is rib fracture. If the patient experiences pain on inspiration following external cardiac massage, this should be reported immediately.

Eating and drinking

During cardiac arrest and resuscitation procedures a patient may vomit, and create problems for the maintenance of a clear airway. When appropriate sheets and clothing should be changed as soon as possible for the patient's comfort and dignity.

Relevance to the
activities of living
continued

Eliminating

There may be incontinence of urine or faeces immediately following a cardiac arrest, which adds to the patient's distress, and sheets and clothing should be changed as soon as possible for his comfort and dignity.

Personal cleansing and dressing

As cardiopulmonary resuscitation is an emergency procedure when immediate exposure of the patient's chest and limbs is required, some damage to the patient's clothing may occur, and this should be explained to the patient after he has had a chance to rest.

Immediately following successful resuscitation the patient will require nursing intervention related to this activity of living to ensure that he is as comfortable as possible.

Sleeping

Following resuscitation and regaining consciousness a patient may have difficulty in resuming his normal sleep pattern due to the fear of suffering a further cardiac arrest, and the nurse should take appropriate measures to help to induce sleep.

Dying

As cardiac arrest is an emergency and may not be reversible, the patient's next of kin may suddenly have to be told of their relative's death and will display any of the many grief reactions, so the nurse's empathy and support are required.

Suggested reading

Chamberlain D 1989 Advanced life support. British Medical Journal 299(6696) August 12: 446–448

Ellis F 1990 Think pink (describes learning of cardiopulmonary resuscitation). Nursing Times 86(34) August 22: 52–53

Evans A 1989 To resuscitate or not. Surgical Nurse 2(1) February: 9–11

Ferguson A 1990 Cardiopulmonary resuscitation – a teaching guide. Nurse Education Today 10: 50–53

Marsden A 1989 Basic life support. British Medical Journal 299(6696) August 12: 442–445

Newbold D 1987 The physiology of cardiac massage. Nursing Times 83(25) June 24: 59–62

Newbold D 1987 External chest compression. Nursing Times 83(26) July 1: 41–43

Roper N, Logan W, Tierney A 1990 The elements of nursing, 3rd edn. Churchill Livingstone, Edinburgh, ch 8

Stewart K, Raj G 1989 A matter of life and death. Nursing Times 85(35) August 30: 27–29

Thom A 1988 Who decides? (opinions about the decision to resuscitate). Nursing Times 85(2) January 11: 35–37

Thompson D, Hopkins S 1987 Making sense of defibrillation. Nursing Times 83(49) December 9: 54–55

Wynne G 1990 Revised guidelines for life support. Nursing Times 86(3) January 17: 70–75

Wynne G, Kirby S, Cordinglya A 1990 No breathing ... no pulse. Professional Nurse 5(10) July: 510–513

Section 4

Eating and Drinking

Feeding a Dependent Patient

Objectives
By the end of this section you should know how to:

- prepare the patient for this nursing practice
- collect and prepare the equipment
- carry out feeding a dependent patient

Related information
Revision of the anatomy and physiology of the mouth and oesophagus with special reference to the physical acts of mastication and swallowing.

Some indications for the feeding of a dependent patient

- to assist a patient who is unable to use his upper limbs due to paralysis or serious illness
- to assist a patient who has lost upper limb coordination due to a physical or mental disease
- to assist a patient who has recently lost his eyesight
- to assist a patient who has an injury around the mouth

Equipment
Feeding utensils such as a fork, knife, spoon, drinking cup with a spout or a cup with angled straw
Disposable napkin or paper towel
Diet as ordered by the patient
Trolley or tray for equipment
Receptacle for soiled disposables

Guidelines for this nursing practice

- explain the nursing practice to the patient and gain his consent and cooperation
- collect and prepare the equipment
- help the patient into a comfortable position
- observe the patient throughout this activity
- wash the hands
- keep the food not being eaten at a suitable temperature
- remind the patient of his ordered menu
- where possible the nurse should sit down while feeding the patient so that this is made an enjoyable social occasion

- ask the patient which food he wishes to eat first
- offer the food to the patient at a rate set by the patient
- place the spoon or fork accurately into the patient's mouth
- offer sips of fluid during the meal
- discontinue feeding when asked by the patient
- ensure the patient is left feeling as comfortable as possible
- dispose of equipment safely
- document the nursing practice appropriately, monitor after-effects and report abnormal findings immediately

Feeding a Dependent Patient

Maintaining a safe environment

All equipment should be clean and all precautions be taken to prevent cross-infection. The nurse should wash her hands before commencing and on completion of the nursing practice.

The nurse will require to check the temperature of the food with the patient to prevent a burn of the mouth, lips or tongue.

Communicating

The patient should be assisted to choose and order his own food from the hospital menu. Eating is a pleasant social occasion for most people, therefore the nurse must help to maintain the atmosphere.

The patient should be shown the food to be eaten as this will assist in the digestion of the food.

A blind patient should be told what food to expect, to avoid the shock of an unexpected taste.

Breathing

The nurse should observe the patient for difficulty in swallowing which may precede choking. Placing the spoon or fork too far back in the patient's mouth may produce gagging or choking.

Eating and drinking

Drinks of fluid will assist a patient to swallow food and also rid the mouth of the taste of one food prior to a different taste.

The patient should be given the choice of feeding utensil to be used when appropriate. Some patients do not like to use a feeding cup with spout, but prefer a straw used with a cup or glass.

A patient who has a motor or sensory loss of one side of the face will need to be fed on the unaffected side of the mouth. The nurse should check that food does not accumulate in the cheek of the affected side.

When possible the patient should be assisted to put the food into his own mouth as this may help him to feel less dependent on the nurse.

Drinks and other foods such as a piece of fruit or a sweet should be offered at frequent intervals other than meal times.

Relatives of the patient may wish to assist the patient in taking food. This should be encouraged as it is of great psychological benefit both to the patient and the relatives.

Personal cleansing and dressing

On ending the meal, the nurse should ask the patient if he wishes his face to be washed and if mouth hygiene is desired.

Suggested reading   Baughen R 1989 Hospital food – a literature review. Surgical Nurse 2(3) June: 18–22
Cabell C 1990 Regaining a basic pleasure (describes care to regain the swallowing
     reflex). Nursing Times 86(47) November 21: 27–29
Committee on Medical Aspects of Food Policy 1984 Diet and cardiovascular disease.
     HMSO, London
Janes E 1980 Hospital food: how well does it go down? Nursing 1(11) March: 487–489
National Advisory Committee on Nutrition Education 1983 A discussion paper on
     proposals of nutritional guidelines for health education in Britain. Health Education
     Council, London
Roper N, Logan W, Tierney A 1990 The elements of nursing, 3rd edn. Churchill
     Livingstone, Edinburgh, pp 154–156, 160–164
Sadler C 1990 Sandwich course (discusses the axing of hot evening meals). Nursing
     Times 86(36) September 5: 19
Sanford J 1987 Making meals a pleasure. Nursing Times 83(6) February 11: 31–32
Scott D 1986 Time and patience. Nursing Times 82(32) August 6: 36–37
Taylor M 1985 Care about food: 'Nurse I'm starving'. Nursing Times 81(23) June 5: 31
Tredger J 1982 Feeding the patient. Nursing 2(4) August: 92–93
Westland M 1982 The human diet. Nursing 2(4) August: 89–91

Gastric Aspiration

Objectives

By the end of this section you should know how to:

- prepare the patient for this nursing practice
- collect and prepare the equipment
- pass a nasogastric tube
- aspirate the stomach contents

Related information

Revision of the anatomy and physiology of the nose, pharynx, oesophagus and stomach.

Some indications for gastric aspiration

Gastric aspiration is a means of keeping the stomach empty of contents by passing a tube into it and applying some form of suction. It is usually performed in the following circumstances:

- obstruction of the bowel
- paralytic ileus
- preoperatively for gastric or some abdominal surgery, e.g. perforated gastric ulcer, oesophageal and gastric varices
- postoperatively, e.g. partial gastrectomy, cholecystectomy

Equipment

Trolley
Protective covering for the patient
Denture dish
Equipment for cleaning nostrils, if required
Nasogastric tube
Lubricant, e.g. iced water, water-soluble jelly
Catheter-tipped syringe
Receiver for aspirated fluid
Receptacle for soiled disposables
Litmus paper
Hypoallergenic tape
Stethoscope
Suction pump

The size of tube selection depends on the size and age of the patient. The most commonly used sizes for the average adult are 14 and 16 FG

Guidelines for this nursing practice

- explain the nursing practice to the patient and gain his consent and cooperation

- collect and prepare the equipment

- ensure the patient's privacy

- help the patient into as comfortable and relaxed a position as possible, sitting upright either in bed or on a chair

- observe the patient throughout this activity

- measure approximately the distance from the patient's nose to his stomach and mark it on the nasogastric tube

- remove the patient's dentures, if present, and place in a labelled container

- ask the patient to blow his nose and sniff each nostril in turn, or clean the nostrils if necessary

- ask the patient if he has any nasal defect or tenderness and change to the other nostril if the first nostril appears blocked. Do not use great force

- ask the patient to relax as much as possible while the tube is being passed

- insert the tube and slide it gently but firmly inwards and backwards along the floor of the nose to the nasopharynx

- encourage the patient to swallow and breathe through his mouth when the tube reaches the pharynx, keeping the chin down and the head forward in order to assist the passage of the tube

- carry out a test to confirm that the tube is in the stomach, when it has reached the measured distance

- secure the tube with tape when there is confirmation that it is in the stomach (Fig. 4.1)

- aspirate the stomach contents. Either continuous or intermittent aspiration will be ordered by the medical practitioner

- ensure that the patient is left feeling as comfortable as possible

- dispose of the equipment safely

- document this nursing practice appropriately, monitor after-effects and report abnormal findings immediately

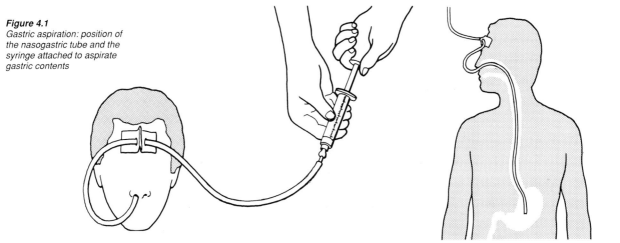

Figure 4.1
Gastric aspiration: position of the nasogastric tube and the syringe attached to aspirate gastric contents

Guidelines for this nursing practice *continued*

The recommended test to confirm the presence of the tube in the stomach is to aspirate some of the stomach contents using a catheter-tipped syringe and test them for acidity with litmus paper. If the aspirate is from the stomach the acidity will turn blue litmus paper pink. If it is not possible to aspirate sufficient stomach contents for testing, some air can be blown into the stomach through the syringe, while a second nurse listens with a stethoscope for the noise of the bubbles of air entering the stomach.

Continuous aspiration can be carried out by some form of pump; the recommended suction pressure is 20–25 mmHg. Less pressure is ineffective and greater pressure can damage the lining of the stomach. Sometimes, usually postoperatively, a drainage bag and tubing may be attached to the end of the nasogastric tube. If the drainage bag is placed lower than the patient's stomach, the stomach contents will siphon into the bag.

Intermittent aspiration can be by pump or catheter-tipped syringe.Between aspirations, a clean spigot should be inserted in the end of the tube.

Relevance to the activities of living

Maintaining a safe environment

Although this does not require aseptic technique, all the equipment should be clean or disposable and the nurse should wash her hands before commencing and on completion of this practice.

In order to prevent damage to the relevant respiratory and alimentary mucosa it is the nurse's duty to ensure that the tube is in the correct position and that the correct pressure of suction is applied.

Communicating

Communication, especially verbal, may be restricted. A pad of paper and pen may be helpful to the patient.

Breathing

The presence of a nasogastric tube may affect the rate and quality of respiration.

It may also cause dryness and irritation in the patient's nose, so a lubricant at, and just beyond, the nasal orifice may reduce discomfort.

Mouth breathing often occurs because of the size of the tube, so oral hygiene should be maintained.

Eating and drinking

When nasogastric aspiration is in progress the patient will not be permitted any solid food by mouth but restricted fluids may be allowed.

Personal cleansing and dressing

The presence of the tube may predispose to dry mucous membranes in the nose and mouth, so frequent oral and nasal hygiene will be necessary.

Mobilising

Mobility may be limited because of the presence of the nasogastric tube and possible connection to suction apparatus.

Expressing sexuality

When a nasogastric tube is in position, the patient may be concerned about his appearance and if it remains in position for a length of time, he may be affected by his altered body image.

Sleeping

Sleep may be affected by the presence of the tube. The patient's sleeping pattern may also be interrupted if intermittent suction is being performed.

Suggested reading

Creach T 1988 Nasogastric warnings. Nursing Times 84(7) February 17: 46–47
Hamilton H (ed) 1985 Nurse's reference library – procedures. Springhouse Corporation, Pennsylvania, pp 540–546
Keane C 1986 Essentials of medical–surgical nursing, 2nd edn. W.B. Saunders, Philadelphia, pp 410–412
Long B, Phipps W 1985 Essentials of medical–surgical nursing – a nursing process approach. C.V. Mosby, St Louis, pp 889–893
Price B 1989 Making sense of nasogastric intubation. Nursing Times 85(13) March 29: 50–52

Enteral Feeding

There are three parts to this section:

1 Enteral feeding via a nasogastric tube and funnel
2 Enteral feeding via a continuous drip system
3 Enteral feeding via a gastrostomy tube

The concluding subsection, 'Relevance to the activities of living', refers to the three practices collectively.

Objectives

By the end of this section you should know how to:

- prepare the patient for this nursing practice
- collect and prepare the equipment
- describe the principles of enteral feeding
- outline some of the problems of enteral feeding

Related information

Revision of the anatomy and physiology of the gastrointestinal tract.

Revision of the nutritional requirements of the human body.

Some indications for enteral feeding

Enteral feeding is the introduction of the daily nutritional requirements, in liquid form, directly into a patient's stomach by means of a tube. The tube may be inserted through the nostril and passed down into the stomach or it may be introduced directly into the stomach by a surgical incision made in the abdominal wall.

It may be performed in the following circumstances:

- obstruction of oesophagus, e.g. neoplasm
- loss of swallowing reflex
- oesophageal fistula
- preoperative preparation of malnourished patients
- postoperatively for patients who have had some oral surgery or oesophageal surgery
- some unconscious patients
- patients who have severe burns
- during radiotherapy treatment

Enteral feeding can be administered in several ways. It may be administered through a funnel and nasogastric tube or continuously through a fine tube, e.g. Clinifeed, with its own administration set and container for the feed; this administers the feed at a set rate. Enteral feeding may also be given through a tube via a surgical opening in the abdominal wall into the stomach, duodenum or jejunum.

1   ENTERAL FEEDING VIA A NASOGASTRIC TUBE AND FUNNEL

Equipment

As for Gastric aspiration (see p. 162)

and

Appropriate feed in jug at room temperature
Funnel
Water
Receptacle for soiled disposables

Guidelines for this nursing practice

- follow guidelines for gastric aspiration including test to confirm the presence of the tube in the patient's stomach (see p. 164)

- observe the patient throughout this activity

- connect the funnel to the end of the tube

- pour a little water through the funnel and tube

- pour some feed into the funnel before all the water has run through

- determine the rate of flow of the feed by the level at which the funnel is held. The higher the funnel is held, the faster the rate of flow will be. The feed should be administered at a fairly slow, steady rate to avoid uncomfortable stomach distension

- pour some water through the tube to clear it, at the end of the feed

- ensure that the patient is left feeling as comfortable as possible

- dispose of the equipment

- record appropriately the time, type and amount of the feed, monitor after-effects and report abnormal findings immediately

The wide-bore rubber or PVC tubes used for this type of feeding can damage the mucosa if left in position for more than 24 hours. This form of feeding has been found to cause more problems and take more nursing time than the continuous drip system. It can cause severe gastrointestinal distension and diarrhoea and vomiting, because of the large amounts of food being poured into the stomach fairly rapidly. It is also easy for patients to become dehydrated when receiving this form of feeding because the nursing staff may cut down on the amount of fluid being given in order to avoid overloading the stomach.

2   ENTERAL FEEDING VIA A CONTINUOUS DRIP SYSTEM

Equipment

Clinifeed tube and introducer
Lubricant
Hypoallergenic tape
Container with prepared feed
Clinifeed administration set (Fig. 4.2)
Intravenous infusion stand
Receptacle for soiled disposables

Figure 4.2
Enteral feeding: nasogastric
continuous drip system

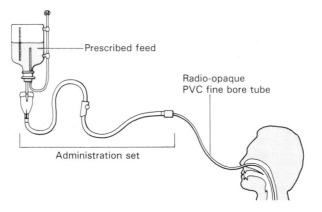

Prescribed feed

Radio-opaque
PVC fine bore tube

Administration set

Guidelines for this nursing practice

- help to explain the nursing practice to the patient and gain his consent and cooperation

- collect and prepare the equipment

- observe the patient throughout this activity

- assist the qualified practitioner to insert the Clinifeed tube and then remove the introducer

- before commencing the feed an X-ray to confirm the position of the tube is necessary, as the lumen is too narrow to allow the usual tests to be carried out

- attach the prepared feed in the container to the infusion stand

- join the administration set to the container and allow the feed to run through to the end of the set before it is connected to the Clinifeed tube so that as little air as possible is introduced to the patient's stomach

- adjust the flow rate as required

- run through some water at the end of the feed to clear the tube

- ensure that the patient is left feeling as comfortable as possible

- record appropriately the time, amount and type of feed given, monitor after-effects and report abnormal findings immediately

Narrow-bore tubes for continuous enteral feeding are a fairly recent innovation. They are made of silicone or polyurethane, with diameters from 1–3 mm. They are more comfortable for the patient than the wide-bore tube and less likely to cause ulceration or erosion of the mucosa. They do, however, become blocked more easily and it is almost impossible to clear them by aspiration.

3 ENTERAL FEEDING VIA A GASTROSTOMY TUBE

Equipment

Funnel and clamp
Water
Prepared feed in container
Sterile spigot
Sterile dressings pack
Water-based antiseptic
Hypoallergenic tape
Receptacle for soiled disposables

Guidelines for this nursing practice

- explain the nursing practice to the patient and gain his consent and cooperation

- assist the patient into a suitable position for easy access to the gastrostomy site

- observe the patient throughout this activity

- collect and prepare the equipment

- connect the funnel and clamp to the gastrostomy tube

- pour a little water through the tube to ensure it is clear

- clamp the tube before all the water has run through so that unnecessary air is not introduced into the stomach as this can cause pain and distension

- start pouring the prepared feed slowly into the stomach by pouring an amount into the funnel and releasing the clamp on the tube (Fig. 4.3). The rate of flow can be adjusted by lowering or raising the funnel

- flush the tube through with water when all the prepared feed has been given

- remove the clamp and funnel and put a clean spigot in the end of the tube

- clean and redress the gastrostomy site using an aseptic technique

- ensure that the patient is left feeling as comfortable as possible

- dispose of the equipment safely

- record appropriately the time, amount and type of feed, monitor after-effects and report abnormal findings immediately

Figure 4.3
Enteral feeding via a gastrostomy tube

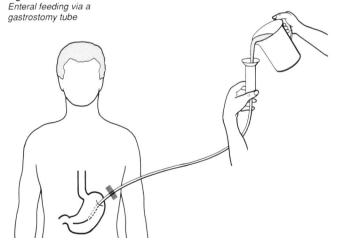

Enteral Feeding

Relevance to the activities of living

Maintaining a safe environment

Although aseptic technique is not necessary when administering enteral feeding, a good standard of hygiene must be maintained to prevent the patient developing a gastrointestinal infection. A strict aseptic technique is necessary when redressing the gastrostomy site to help prevent the wound becoming infected.

No feed should be administered until the nurse has checked that the nasogastric tube is in the correct position.

Eating and drinking

The patient may be allowed a small amount of liquid orally. This can help to stimulate secretion of some of the digestive juices. It is necessary to ensure that the patient receives an adequate amount of fluid in 24 hours and all the essential nutrients.

Nausea can be a problem and is often caused by the feed being administered too rapidly. The continuous drip system helps to overcome this.

Eliminating

Diarrhoea can be a problem and is usually caused by too rapid feeding or administering a feed which is too concentrated. A feed contaminated by pathogens would also result in diarrhoea.

Personal cleansing and dressing

Frequent oral hygiene should be offered to the patient receiving enteral feeding because his lips, tongue and the mucosa of his mouth rapidly become dry and cracked if no fluid is passing over them.

Sleeping

Patients may prefer to receive their food by the continuous drip system while they are asleep at night. This allows them more freedom of movement during the day.

Suggested reading

Anderson B 1986 Tube feeding: is diarrhoea inevitable? American Journal of Nursing 86(6) June: 704–706

Bladen L 1986 Enteral nutrition. Nursing 3(8) August: 281–285

Boore J, Champion R, Ferguson M (eds) 1987 Nursing the physically ill adult. Churchill Livingstone, Edinburgh, ch 14

Gibbs J 1983 Bacterial contamination of nasogastric feeds. Nursing Times Journal of Infection Control 79(7) February 16: 41–47

Goodinson S 1986 Assessment of nutritional states. Nursing 3(7) July: 252–258

Holmes S 1986 Fundamentals of nutrition. Nursing 3(7) July: 235–239

Janes E 1982 Nursing aspects of tube feeding. Nursing 2(4) August: 101–104

Roper N, Logan W, Tierney A 1990 The elements of nursing, 3rd edn. Churchill Livingstone, Edinburgh, pp 166–167

Taylor S 1988 A guide to nasogastric feeding. Professional Nurse 3(11) August: 439–443

Taylor S 1988 A guide to nasogastric feeding equipment. Professional Nurse 4(2) November: 91–93

Westland M 1982 The human diet. Nursing 2(4) August: 89–91

Gastric Lavage

Objectives

By the end of this section you should know how to:

- prepare the patient for this procedure
- collect and prepare the equipment
- assist with the procedure of gastric lavage

Related information

Revision of the anatomy and physiology of the upper alimentary tract.

Review of health authority policy on gastric lavage.

Some indications for gastric lavage

Gastric lavage involves introducing a wide-bore tube into the stomach and washing out the contents by pouring in and siphoning off a prescribed solution. It is sometimes necessary:

- to obtain a specimen of gastric contents
- to remove harmful substances swallowed accidentally or deliberately

Outline of the procedure

Health authority policies vary on who is qualified to perform a gastric lavage. As a general rule, medical practitioners carry it out on unconscious patients and specially trained nursing staff in accident and emergency units can carry it out on conscious patients.

The tube will be passed through the patient's mouth and if he is conscious he will be asked to swallow it. Once the marked length on the tube has been reached, one of the tests to check that the tube is in the stomach, described in the section on gastric aspiration, will be performed (see p. 164). Some of the stomach contents may then be aspirated to obtain specimens for analysis. The tubing and funnel are attached to the stomach tube and 150–300 ml of solution are poured into the stomach. If the stomach is overfilled some of the contents may be forced through the pylorus. The funnel is then lowered and the gastric contents siphoned into the bucket. The lavage will be repeated until the return flow is relatively clear. The tube is pinched when it is being withdrawn to maintain suction and prevent stimulation of the vomiting reflex.

Equipment

As for gastric aspiration (see p. 162), but the tube should have a much larger lumen (e.g. 30 gauge Jacques stomach tube)

and

Mouth gag
Funnel and connecting tubing
Bucket for aspirate
Tap water or prescribed solution
Sterile containers appropriately labelled for specimens of aspirate
Laboratory form
Plastic specimen bag for transportation

Guidelines for this nursing practice

- collect and prepare the required equipment
- explain the procedure to the patient if possible and try to gain his consent and cooperation
- ensure the patient's privacy
- remove dentures if appropriate and place in a labelled container
- measure the approximate distance between mouth and stomach and mark tube
- help the patient into the position requested by the person passing the tube
- observe the patient throughout this activity
- lubricate the end of the tube
- assist the person passing the tube
- ensure the patient is left feeling as comfortable as possible
- dispose of the equipment safely
- document this procedure appropriately, monitor after-effects, and report abnormal findings immediately
- dispatch labelled specimens and completed forms to the laboratory

Relevance to the activities of living

Maintaining a safe environment

Although this does not require aseptic technique, all the equipment should be clean or disposable and the nurse should wash her hands before commencing and on completion of the procedure.

The safety of the patient is a prime consideration, so because of the obvious risks only a medical practitioner or a suitably qualified member of the nursing staff will carry out this procedure. If the patient is unconscious, a medical practitioner will carry out the procedure. For the safe transport of specimens see Specimen collection, p. 198.

Breathing

If the patient is unconscious a nasotracheal tube will be passed before the stomach tube to ensure the maintenance of a clear airway.

Eating and drinking

The tube used for this procedure has a large lumen and cannot be left in position for a long period as it will cause tissue irritation and damage.

Sleeping

As mentioned already this procedure may be carried out on an unconscious patient and so all reasonable precautions must be taken for the patient's safety. He should be placed in the recovery position and observed constantly. His vital signs should be monitored.

Suggested reading

Bradley D 1984 Accident and emergency nursing. Baillière Tindall, London, pp 227–233
Johnstone F 1987 Self poisoning. Nursing 3(16) April: 602–608
Luckmann J, Sorensen K 1980 Medical–surgical nursing. W.B. Saunders, Philadelphia, pp 2203–2205

Parenteral Nutrition

Objectives

By the end of this section you should know how to:

- prepare the patient for this procedure
- collect and prepare the equipment
- assist the medical practitioner with the insertion of a central venous catheter
- maintain an infusion of parenteral nutrition for a period of time

Related information

Revision of the anatomy and physiology of the cardiopulmonary system with special reference to the circulation of the blood, and the veins of the neck and upper thorax.

Revision of intravenous therapy (see p. 104).

Revision of aseptic technique (see p. 26).

Review of health authority policy regarding parenteral nutrition.

Some indications for parenteral nutrition

Parenteral nutrition is the intravenous infusion of essential nutrients for patients who are unable to maintain an adequate nutritional intake by the oral or nasogastric route. It may be indicated:

- for patients who have had surgery involving major resection of the intestine
- for patients who have extensive inflammatory disease of the alimentary system
- for patients who have malabsorption problems
- for patients who have severe nausea and vomiting, e.g. following chemotherapy for malignant disease

Total parenteral nutrition (TPN) is the term used when all the patient's nutritional requirements are given by intravenous infusion. Parenteral nutrition may be given as a supplement to nasogastric or oral feeding.

Outline of the procedure

Ideally this procedure should be performed in theatre. If the procedure is performed in the ward, it should take place in the treatment room.

The insertion of the intravenous catheter used for an infusion of parenteral nutrition is performed by a medical practitioner using aseptic technique. A cap and theatre mask are worn. Having washed his hands the medical practitioner dons a theatre gown and gloves, and prepares the sterile equipment on the trolley, maintaining asepsis. When the patient is in the correct position, sterile drapes are placed round the area of the access site. A local anaesthetic may be administered. The skin area of the access site is cleansed prior to the insertion of an intravenous catheter through the subclavian or the internal jugular vein to allow the tip of the catheter to lie in the superior vena cava. A flow of prescribed infusion fluid is established, and the distal end of the catheter is stitched in position. The access site is covered with a sterile dressing (see central venous pressure, p. 124).

Occasionally a catheter will be tunnelled subcutaneously so that the entry site to the vein is separated from the skin entry site to reduce the risk of infection. This is performed when long-term parenteral nutrition is envisaged.

The concentration of the nutrients is irritant to peripheral vessels, and could cause damage to peripheral veins, so parenteral nutrition should always be infused through a central venous catheter. The infusion fluid enters the circulation at the superior vena cava, is rapidly diluted by the volume of blood entering the heart, and quickly distributed by the circulation of the blood thus reducing any problems of irritation to the vessels involved.

The position of the patient is important during this procedure, and is dependent on the choice of entry site for catheterisation. There are three main entry sites:

The subclavian vein: The patient lies supine with no pillow, and the neck is extended. The head of the bed is lowered by 10°.

The internal jugular vein: The patient lies supine with no pillow, and the neck is extended. The head is rotated away from the site of entry, and well supported in position. The head of the bed is lowered by 10°. This position is important to prevent the development of an air embolus.

The median cephalic vein: The patient lies supine. The chosen arm is extended with the palm upwards and the elbow supported.

Equipment

As for intravenous infusion (see p. 104).

Additional equipment

Theatre cap and mask

Sterile gown

Sterile gloves

Sterile minor operation pack or sterile drape and towels

Waterproof protection for the bed

Alcohol-based lotion for cleansing the skin

Prescribed infusion fluid for parenteral nutrition

Appropriate sterile catheter depending on the site of entry used, e.g. Hickman catheter, double or triple lumen catheter

Sterile needles and black silk sutures

ECG monitoring equipment if required

Volumetric infusion pump, e.g. IMED infusion pumps Nos. 922, 960, 965

Cassette for priming infusion pump

Dark bag for excluding light from prepared infusion fluid

Infusion fluid for parenteral nutrition

This will be prescribed by the medical practitioner for each 24-hour period dependent on the patient's nutritional needs and related blood chemistry. A combination of nutrients will be used to give a balanced intake, and vitamins and trace elements will be included in the prescription.

In areas where pharmacy services are available the intravenous feeding regimen is prepared as prescribed for each patient in 2 or 3 litre bags under laminar flow conditions every 24 hours. Everything for parenteral nutrition, including vitamins and trace elements, is added at one time. This reduces the risk of infection which might occur when an infusion of several different fluids in separate containers is prescribed and a series of taps, or Y connectors, are needed for the infusion.

A combination of the following intravenous fluids may be prescribed. All are available in 500 ml containers (see current pharmaceutical literature).

- carbohydrates, e.g. dextrose 20%
- fats, e.g. Intralipid 10%, Intralipid 20%
- proteins, e.g. Vamin 14 EF, Vamin 18 EF

Many other products are available and the choice will depend on the patient's needs and the medical practitioner's preference.

In addition the following may be added:

- vitamins, e.g. Multibionta

NOTE: Some vitamins are destroyed by sunlight; if added to a 24-hour parenteral infusion the container must be covered by a dark bag to exclude any light.

- electrolytes, e.g. potassium, phosphates
- trace elements, e.g. zinc, magnesium

Hickman catheter

This intravenous catheter may be chosen by the medical practitioner for a parenteral infusion which is needed over a period of weeks. This radio-opaque silastic catheter has a small sponge-like Dacron cuff at the distal end. The line is tunnelled subcutaneously and the cuff helps to retain the line in position as fibrous tissue forms round it.

This type of catheter is also used for infusions of intravenous cytotoxic medications which are prescribed over a long period, and are not suitable for a peripheral infusion because of their irritant properties.

Volumetric infusion pumps

Parenteral nutrition should be infused by a continuous volumetric infusion pump. This ensures that a steady flow of prescribed nutrients is infused at a rate suitable for the patient's metabolism. If a pump is unavailable, a burette administration set should be used. Infusion pumps are primed with a special cassette, and introduced into the infusion circuit between the administration set from the infusion fluid, and the infusion catheter (Fig. 4.4). There are clear manufacturer's instructions for all infusion pumps which should be followed when setting up infusions.

Infusion pumps can be set to give an hourly flow rate of 1–999 ml per hour. All pumps are fitted with alarm systems which will monitor any occlusion of the lines, air bubbles and completion of the available fluid. Recent equipment has a digital read-out of details of the infusion, and the alarm system. New equipment for controlled administration of intravenous infusion is being developed continually. There are different types of infusion pumps and gravity-feed infusion sets on the market, and the choice for use may depend on health authority policy.

Figure 4.4
Parenteral nutrition:
equipment for priming the
volumetric infusion pump

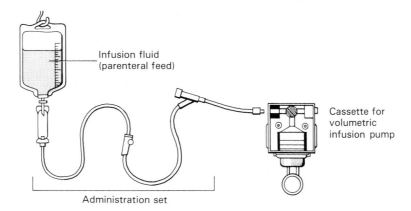

Infusion fluid
(parenteral feed)

Cassette for
volumetric
infusion pump

Administration set

Guidelines for this nursing practice

- help to explain the procedure to the patient and gain his consent and cooperation
- ensure the patient's privacy
- collect and prepare the equipment
- check the prescribed intravenous fluid for parenteral nutrition
- prime the equipment (see Intravenous infusion, p. 104)
- help the patient into the appropriate position, depending on the site of entry used for the insertion of the central venous catheter
- observe the patient throughout this activity
- adjust the tilt of the bed to lower the patient's head if necessary
- remain with the patient and help maintain his position
- assist the medical practitioner as required

- commence the infusion of parenteral nutrition at the prescribed rate once the catheter is in position and the sterile dressing is applied to the access site (see Central venous pressure, p. 124)
- cover the infusion with a dark bag to protect any vitamins from light, which may cause deterioration
- ensure that the patient is left feeling as comfortable as possible
- maintain the infusion as prescribed by dialling the required number of ml per hour on the infusion pump (see manufacturer's instructions) or by filling the burette chamber hourly with the prescribed volume of fluid
- dispose of the equipment safely
- document the nursing practice appropriately, monitor after-effects and report abnormal findings immediately

Relevance to the activities of living

Maintaining a safe environment

All precautions and observations for the prevention of infection should be maintained.

The whole infusion and the administration set should be changed every 24 hours, maintaining asepsis.

The lines should be observed for air bubbles and all the connections checked regularly and the lines supported to prevent any disconnection, in order to help prevent the development of an air embolus.

The alarm systems of the infusion pumps should be familiar to the staff using the equipment, and appropriate action taken when they are activated.

The nurse may help with patient education regarding maintaining a safe environment. Learning aseptic technique of wound cleaning and dressing will allow some independence for patients discharged home with long-term TPN.

Breathing

The respirations should be observed, and all the vital signs recorded 4-hourly or as frequently as necessary. Breathlessness accompanied by a moist cough and frothy sputum may indicate pulmonary oedema due to circulatory overload. Any abnormalities should be reported so that the rate of the prescribed infusion can be adjusted (see Intravenous infusion, p. 104).

A rare complication would be the development of a pneumothorax. This is more likely to occur at the time of insertion of the catheter. Any sudden change in the patient's general condition or respiratory function should be reported.

Eating and drinking

Accurate fluid balance recordings should be maintained. Fluid intake should be recorded as frequently as necessary, depending on the patient's condition hourly, 2-hourly or 4-hourly. Details of IV nutrients infused should also be recorded.

Initially the patient's blood sugar levels may be monitored regularly while parenteral nutrition is in progress. The results will indicate the patient's ability to metabolise the nutrients infused.

Ward urinalysis should be performed for sugar and acetone 4-hourly.

Blood sugar estimation using BM sticks or Dextrostix should be performed 4-hourly or as ordered.

Occasionally a continuous infusion of insulin is prescribed for patients who need a large calorie intake but whose metabolism is temporarily deficient. This may occur when a patient has severe trauma, burns or scalds.

Some patients may have long-term Total Parenteral Nutrition (TPN) and be discharged home with a continuous, or intermittent infusion. Patient education, and the help and support of the primary health care team may allow the patient to become independent in the administration of his own TPN.

A patient receiving parenteral nutrition has little or nothing to eat or drink by mouth. Frequent oral hygiene should be performed to maintain a healthy oral mucosa until a normal diet is resumed. With appropriate health education, patients with long-term TPN may be helped to become independent in keeping their oral mucosa healthy.

Eliminating

Fluid output should be recorded to maintain accurate fluid balance charts and help monitor renal function.

Help may be needed when using a commode to help support the infusion lines and prevent any disconnection.

Relevance to the
activities of living
continued

Personal cleansing and dressing

Light comfortable clothing will allow access to the infusion site, and the reason for this should be explained to the patient. Help may be needed with washing and showering. Some patients may be discharged home with TPN, and help given by carers and the district nurse.

Expressing sexuality

Having a continuous infusion, and a long-term central line will give an altered body image. Perceptive and supportive nursing care and good communication skills will help to alleviate this.

At home, adaptation of normal clothes, as well as counselling and help from the primary health care team will enable normal activities to resume as far as possible, restoring the patient's self esteem.

Mobilising

In some instances parenteral nutrition may continue when the patient is up and about in the ward and staff can help the patient to take his infusion with him. A light mobile pole and supportive explanations in relation to maintaining a safe environment will give the patient confidence to be more independent and visit other patients or the television room, as his condition allows. Occasionally patients may be discharged home while still receiving parenteral nutrition; with supervision and counselling from the primary health care team they can resume many normal activities.

Sleeping

The normal sleeping position may have to be adapted to accommodate the infusion lines, and the patient helped into a comfortable position.

Patients on long-term home TPN (HTPN) may choose the times of their nutritional infusion period. This may be given overnight, so that a more normal lifestyle may be resumed during the day.

Suggested reading

Boore J et al (eds) 1987 Nursing the physically ill adult. Churchill Livingstone, Edinburgh, Ch 14

Clarke R 1990 A cost effective system for TPN. Nursing Times 86(31) August 1: 65–68

Dewar B 1986 Total parenteral nutrition at home. Nursing Times 82(28) July 9: 35–38

Finnigan S et al 1989 When eating is impossible. TPN in maintaining nutritional state. Professional Nurse 4(6) March: 271–275

Liston L 1987 Paediatric HTPN. A father's view. Intensive Therapy & Clinical Monitoring November/December: 186, 189, 196

Michie B 1988 Total parenteral nutrition. Nursing Times 84(20) May 18: 46–47

Roper N, Logan W, Tierney A 1990 The elements of nursing, 3rd edn. Churchill Livingstone, Edinburgh, pp 164–176

Blood Glucose Estimation

Objectives

By the end of this section you should know how to:

- prepare the patient for this nursing practice
- collect and prepare the equipment
- carry out blood glucose estimation

Related information

Revision of the anatomy and physiology of the endocrine system with special reference to the regulation of blood glucose.

Revision of the manufacturer's information on the reagent strips.

Some indications for blood glucose estimation

Blood glucose estimation is the measurement of the level of blood glucose using a chemical reagent strip:

- to assist in the monitoring of primary diabetes mellitus due to pancreatic disease or other hormone disorders

Equipment

Sterile lancet or pricking device, e.g. Autolet
Cotton wool balls
Blood testing strip, e.g. BM Glycemie 1–44
Glucose meter if available
Disposable gloves
Tray for equipment
Watch with a seconds hand
Receptacle for soiled disposables

Guidelines for this nursing practice

- explain the nursing practice to the patient and obtain his consent and cooperation
- collect and prepare the equipment
- wash the hands
- don disposable gloves
- ensure the patient's privacy
- check the expiry date on the container label
- help the patient into a comfortable position
- observe the patient throughout the activity
- help the patient to wash his hands with soap and warm water and dry thoroughly
- using the lancet or pricking device prick the patient's finger
- gently massage the finger to obtain a drop of blood which must be large enough to cover the reagent pads
- allow the drop of blood to come in contact with the reagent pads without smearing and spreading the blood
- note the time

- apply a clean cotton wool ball to prick site
- after the elapsed time as recommended by the manufacturer, carefully and firmly wipe the blood off the test strip using a clean cotton wool ball
- wipe the reagent pads twice more using a clean piece of cotton wool each time
- allow the second period of time to elapse as recommended by the manufacturer
- compare the colours of the reagent pads with the manufacturer's scale, usually found on the reagent strip container

or

- Place the reagent strip in the recommended glucose meter
- note the result
- dispose of the equipment safely
- ensure the patient is left feeling as comfortable as possible
- document the nursing practice appropriately, monitor after-effects and report abnormal findings immediately

Blood Glucose Estimation

Relevance to the
activities of living

Maintaining a safe environment

All containers of reagent strips when not in use should be stored in a locked cupboard or drawer to comply with health and safety at work regulations. The manufacturer's recommendations for the conditions of storage, technique and use must be observed, otherwise inaccurate results may be obtained from the reagent strips.

The nurse should assess the blood glucose level at the specific time ordered by the medical practitioner.

Contamination of the reagent pads or the patient's blood could lead to inaccurate results. The patient's finger should not be cleansed with an alcohol-saturated wipe as the alcohol would act as a contaminant and cause the skin to harden with constant use. Any reagent strip accidentally contaminated by the nurse or the patient must be discarded.

Clean dry absorbent cotton wool should be used to wipe the reagent strip, as the use of any other material may alter the results of the test.

Glucose meters can be of benefit when noting the results of the blood glucose estimation for both nurse or patient but they are expensive to buy. The meter also requires to be calibrated at regular intervals by trained personnel.

Gloves should be worn when estimating a patient's blood glucose level to prevent cross-infection from blood-borne viral infections such as hepatitis B or HIV (AIDS).

Communicating

Some patients find the finger pricking rather uncomfortable. The automatic pricking devices may help to reduce the discomfort.

The nurse may require to teach a patient to carry out his own blood glucose estimation or other aspects of care and/or treatment. Utilising a skill analysis approach can be of benefit in the teaching process.

Blood glucose levels are measured in mmol/l. The normal range of blood glucose level is between 3.7 mmol/l and no greater than 10 mmol/l after a meal. Hypoglycaemia is the term used to describe an abnormally low blood glucose. Hyperglycaemia descibes an excessively high blood glucose.

The nurse should use her observational skills as the information gained may alert her to the development of a complication which could be fatal, e.g. the development of hypoglycaemic or hyperglycaemic coma.

The results from blood glucose estimation will usually be recorded on a diabetic/insulin chart.

Breathing

Development of tachycardia or palpitation by the patient can be suggestive of hypoglycaemic coma.

Eating and drinking

The most common reason for estimating blood glucose is for diabetes mellitus. A patient will usually be receiving a special diabetic diet which must be closely followed. The patient will require support and education to cope with this change in his eating habits.

Eliminating

Blood glucose estimation is a more accurate assessment of blood glucose level than assessing the level of glucose in urine. Each patient's renal threshold (the level at which the blood glucose spills over into the urine) can vary, therefore measurement of glucose in the urine can be an inaccurate guide to the effectiveness of hormonal control of the glucose level in the body.

Suggested reading

Almond J 1986 Measuring blood glucose levels. Nursing Times 82(41) October 8: 51–54

Ames Division Self blood glucose monitoring, 2nd edn. Bayer Diagnostics UK Limited, Slough (available from Bayer Diagnostics UK Limited, Stoke Court, Stoke Poges, Slough SL2 4LY)

Boore J, Champion R, Ferguson M (eds) 1987 Nursing the physically ill adult. Churchill Livingstone, Edinburgh, pp 493–511

Dunn S 1987 Blood glucose monitoring and learned helplessness. Practical Diabetes 4(3) May/June: 108–110

Ginsburg J, Fink R 1983 Diabetes mellitus. Nursing 2(13) May: 369–378

Heenan A 1990 Blood glucose measurement. Nursing Times 86(4) January 24: 65–68

Newton R 1987 Testing testing ... Nursing Times Community Outlook 83(2) January 14:16–18

Reading S 1986 Blood glucose monitoring – teaching effective techniques. The Professional Nurse 2(2) November: 55–57

Roper N, Logan W, Tierney A 1990 The elements of nursing, 3rd edn. Churchill Livingstone, Edinburgh, pp 164–165

Tsang W, Griffin H 1988 Making sense of blood glucose estimation. Nursing Times 84(25) June 22: 40–41

Liver Biopsy

Objectives

By the end of this section you should know how to:

- prepare the patient for this procedure
- collect and prepare the equipment
- assist the medical practitioner during the procedure
- care for the patient prior to, during and following the procedure

Related information

Revision of the anatomy and physiology of the liver with special reference to the position and the functions of the liver.

Revision of aseptic technique (see p. 26).

Some indications for a liver biopsy

A liver biopsy is the removal of a small piece of liver tissue using a specially designed needle:

- to aid in the diagnosis of a liver disease

Outline of the procedure

Prior to this investigation the patient will have blood samples taken for estimation of bleeding, clotting and prothrombin times. A platelet count, grouping and cross-matching will also be requested by the medical practitioner. A patient who requires a liver biopsy may be suffering from a blood clotting defect which may prevent or defer their investigation. The patient may have some form of sedation prescribed prior to the procedure.

The biopsy will be carried out by a medical practitioner under local anaesthetic using an aseptic technique. The patient should lie in a supine position using one pillow with his right hand under his head. The biopsy needle will be inserted through a stab incision to rest above the surface of the liver. The patient is asked to hold his breath in full expiration as the medical practitioner advances the biopsy needle into the liver then withdraws the needle (Fig. 4.5). The patient can then resume his normal breathing pattern. Pressure should be applied to the biopsy site for 5 minutes using a sterile swab. Once the bleeding has ceased or is minimal the site can be sprayed with a plastic dressing and/or a sterile dry dressing applied.

Equipment

Sterile gloves
Sterile dressings pack
Alcohol-based antiseptic for skin cleansing
Local anaesthetic and equipment for its administration
Sterile disposable scalpel or similar equipment
Sterile liver biopsy needle, e.g. Trucut
Sterile adhesive dressing
Sterile specimen container with preservative appropriately labelled and with a completed laboratory form and plastic specimen bag for transportation
Trolley for equipment
Receptacle for soiled disposables

Guidelines for this nursing practice

- help to explain the procedure to the patient and gain his consent and cooperation
- wash the hands
- give the patient sedation if prescribed
- ensure the patient's privacy
- collect and prepare the equipment and trolley as required
- help the patient into the correct position and ensure that he is as comfortable as possible
- observe the patient throughout this activity
- assist the medical practitioner as necessary during the procedure

- remain with the patient and help maintain his position as required during the biopsy
- help the patient re-position himself onto his right side for 2 hours following the liver biopsy
- ensure that the patient is left feeling as comfortable as possible
- dispose of the equipment safely
- dispatch the labelled specimen to the laboratory immediately with the completed laboratory form
- document the nursing practice appropriately, monitor after-effects, and report any abnormal findings immediately

Figure 4.5
Liver biopsy: method of securing a specimen of tissue
A Introducing a biopsy needle: cannula (outer) and obturator (inner)
B Obtaining tissue specimen by advancing the obturator handle, and pushing the cutting edge of the obturator's specimen notch into the liver tissue
C Withdrawing the obturator handle to enclose the specimen within the cannula, then removing the entire biopsy needle

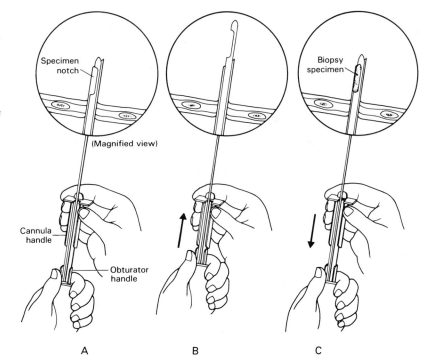

Liver Biopsy

Relevance to the activities of living

Maintaining a safe environment

As this is an invasive procedure all precautions against, and observations to detect, infection should be maintained. Unless a complication arises the adhesive dressing can be removed within 2–3 days following the biopsy.

For safe transportation of the specimen collection see p. 198.

Communicating

An easily understood explanation of the procedure and the aftercare should be given to the patient. This is primarily given by the medical practitioner but the nurse may be required to repeat the explanation.

Requesting the patient to turn his head to the left during the procedure could be helpful in the prevention of an increase in patient anxiety brought about by observing the medical practitioner's actions and the equipment used.

The patient may require a mild analgesic for pain at the biopsy site or referred pain, i.e. shoulder-tip pain. Should the patient complain of severe pain this must be reported to the medical practitioner. This may be a sign of biliary peritonitis, which is known to be a potential complication following liver biopsy.

Breathing

The patient should have frequent recordings of blood pressure, pulse and respiration rates for 24 hours following a liver biopsy. The biopsy site should be observed for continued bleeding or haematoma formation.

A sudden change in the patient's cardiovascular or respiratory function, such as a drop in blood pressure or dyspnoea, must be reported. This may signify injury to other tissues during the biopsy leading to the development of the known complications of haemorrhage or a pneumothorax. The risk of tearing the liver and damaging the lung tissue is greatly reduced if the patient holds his breath in full expiration as the biopsy needle is advanced into the liver.

Mobilising

The patient may remain in bed for the 24 hours following the biopsy, the first 2 hours of the period spent quietly lying on his right side to compress the liver against the chest wall. This will help to reduce the possibility of haemorrhage.

Suggested reading   Booth J 1983 Handbook of investigations. Harper & Row, London, pp 25–27
Brunner L, Suddarth D 1985 The Lippincott manual of medical–surgical nursing,
Volume 2. Harper & Row, London, pp 481–483
Brunner L, Suddarth D 1988 Textbook of medical–surgical nursing, 6th edn. J. B.
Lippincott Company, Philadelphia, pp 860–861
Faulkner A 1985 Nursing – a creative approach. Baillière Tindall, Eastbourne, pp
160–162
Roper N, Logan W, Tierney A 1990 The elements of nursing, 3rd edn. Churchill
Livingstone, Edinburgh, p 164

Section 5

Eliminating

Toileting

Objectives

By the end of this section you should know how to:

- prepare the patient for this nursing practice
- collect and prepare the equipment
- provide facilities for the patient to empty his bladder or bowel

Related information

Revision of the anatomy and physiology of the urinary system, with special reference to micturition.

Revision of the anatomy and physiology of the rectum and anus with special reference to defaecation.

Review of health authority policy regarding disposal of excreta and the control of infection.

Some indications for toileting

Toileting is the provision of appropriate facilities for the patient to micturate or defaecate. This may be a ward toilet, a commode, a bedpan or urinal.

A bedpan, urinal or commode should be provided:

- for patients who are confined to bed or only allowed up for short periods

Assistance to the toilet should be provided:

- for patients who are too frail or immobile to be self-caring in relation to toileting

Equipment

Bedpan, urinal, commode or toilet, as appropriate
Toilet paper
Disposable cover for bedpan or urinal
Measuring jug
Bedpan disposer, e.g. Clinamatic
Bedpan washer for non-disposable equipment
Facilities for hand washing
Facilities for communicating the patient's need for toileting to the nurse, e.g. bell
Receptacle for soiled disposables

Bedpan

For female patients a bedpan may be used for micturition and defaecation. For male patients it may be used for defaecation, and a urinal should be offered at the same time for micturition. Toiletware may be disposable or non-disposable; non-disposable equipment is usually made of stainless steel. Increasingly, disposable equipment is being used.

Disposable bedpan: This should be placed in a rigid bedpan holder and taken to the bedside under a disposable cover. The used bedpan should be flushed in the bedpan disposer according to the manufacturer's instructions. The holder should be washed and dried before storing.

Stainless steel bedpan: This should be warmed under hot water, dried and covered with a disposable cover. The used bedpan should be placed in the bedpan washer and flushed according to the manufacturer's instructions. It should be washed and dried before storing and regular sterilisation should be performed according to health authority policies.

Urinal

This is used for male patients for micturition, and should be covered with a disposable cover when taken to and from the patient. This may also be disposable or non-disposable and, after use, is processed in the same way as a bedpan.

Commode

This is a mobile chair constructed to hold a bedpan which can be taken to the bedside for the patient's use. It may be constructed to transport the patient to the toilet so that the commode seat fits over the toilet seat. Many mechanical lifting aids incorporate a commode seat so that the patient may be taken safely to the ward toilet, or use it as a conventional commode (see manufacturer's instructions).

Guidelines for this nursing practice

Guidelines are given for the provision of a bedpan to a female patient and a urinal to a male patient.

The provision of a bedpan for a female patient

- explain this nursing practice to the patient and gain her consent and cooperation
- ensure that the patient knows how to request a bedpan when needed
- respond immediately to the patient's request for a bedpan
- don a plastic apron
- collect and prepare the bedpan, carrying it to the bedside under a disposable cover
- ensure the patient's privacy
- observe the patient's condition throughout this activity
- help the patient into a comfortable sitting position, supporting her back with pillows
- help the patient to adjust her clothing and expose the buttocks and perineum, removing any appliances
- help to lift the patient's buttocks by placing a hand under the lower lumbar region, using a safe lifting technique. Two nurses may be needed depending on the patient's condition
- slide the bedpan into position with the shaped rim under the patient's buttocks

- adjust the patient's pillows to ensure she is sitting comfortably
- leave the patient to use the bedpan, ensuring privacy
- remain in the vicinity to be available when the patient is ready
- assist with wiping the perineum and/or anus if necessary
- remove the bedpan
- give the patient a bowl to wash her hands
- ensure that the patient is left feeling as comfortable as possible
- observe the contents of the bedpan for any abnormalities; these should be reported and the bedpan saved for inspection
- measure the urine and retain a labelled specimen for ward testing if required (see Testing urine, p. 204)
- dispose of the equipment safely
- document the nursing practice appropriately and report abnormal findings immediately

Guidelines for providing a commode will be in principle the same as those for using a bedpan. Once the prepared and covered commode is taken to the bedside the patient should be helped out of bed to sit on the commode in privacy, and guidelines followed as for a bedpan. Help from one or two nurses may be needed to assist the patient in and out of bed, depending on the patient's condition.

The provision of a urinal for a male patient

- explain this nursing practice and gain the patient's consent and cooperation
- ensure that the patient knows how to request a urinal when needed
- collect and prepare the urinal and take it to the bedside under a disposable cover

- ensure the patient's privacy
- help the patient to place the urinal in position if required
- remain in the vicinity to be available when the patient is ready
- remove the urinal and proceed as for guidelines for providing a bedpan

Relevance to the activities of living

Maintaining a safe environment

To prevent any cross-infection and to maintain adequate standards of hygiene a separate area should be designated for storing and disposal of equipment used for toileting.

Adequate hand washing facilities should be available for both patients and staff in this area and beside the patients' toilets. Good hand washing technique should be maintained to prevent cross-infection. The decision to wear gloves will depend on the individual situation.

All equipment should be washed and dried immediately after use, to prevent any cross-infection.

Plastic aprons should be worn by nursing staff when providing toilet facilities and these should be removed or changed after this nursing practice to prevent cross-infection.

Maintaining the patient's privacy for this activity of living, 'eliminating', sometimes conflicts with the need to maintain the safety of his environment. The nurse must make sure that there is no danger of the patient falling when using a bedpan or commode and that he can be safely left on the ward toilet. The decision about which facilities are used for toileting depends not only on the patient's condition, but also on his orientation and mobility.

Communicating

Good communication skills by the nursing staff can prevent the patient worrying about toilet arrangements. He should be shown the patients' toilets or told how to ask for a bedpan, urinal or commode by the nurse who admits him and the reason for these arrangements should be explained. A bell or other means of requesting assistance should be available as required and requests for toilet facilities should be acted on immediately.

Eliminating is a private activity of living and the nurse's attitude, and non-verbal communication when performing this nursing practice can affect the way the patient accepts the need for particular toilet arrangements.

Eating and drinking

For the patient's own comfort and for the maintenance of personal hygiene, toilet facilities followed by hand washing should be offered before meals for all patients who are not self-caring.

Eliminating

Urine should be measured and the results recorded for patients whose fluid balance is being monitored. Patients who are self-caring, but whose urine is to be measured, should be shown how to place a bedpan over the toilet seat and use that for micturition, so that the nurse can measure the urine. Urine should be observed for any abnormalities and tested as required (see Testing urine, p. 204).

Patient's bowel movements should be recorded, so that any problem of constipation or diarrhoea can be monitored. Any abnormalities noted should be reported immediately (see Specimen of faeces, p. 201).

The patient's condition will dictate whether a bedpan or commode is used when he is confined to bed. However, the stress of using a bedpan may be considerable for some patients, and a commode should be available if possible.

Relevance to the
activities of living
continued

Male patients should be given a urinal for micturition when they require a bedpan or commode for defaecation.

Elderly patients with problems of continence should be helped to use appropriate toilet facilities at frequent intervals, and any request for toileting should be answered immediately, so that the patient may regain adequate bladder control. If the patient is mobile, his bed and chair should be within easy reach of an available toilet to encourage continence. The assistance of one or two nurses may be needed.

Personal cleansing and dressing

The nurse may have to help the patient to wipe or wash and dry the anus, vulval area and perineum following defaecation.

This should always be done so that the wiping or washing is from front to back, away from the urethra, and the paper towel renewed after each wipe. For women particularly it is important that no bacteria from the rectal area reach the urethra, as this may cause a urinary tract infection. Careful perineal toilet should prevent this (see Bed bath, p. 250).

Controlling body temperature

During toileting the patient should be kept warm with adequate clothing and covers, as well as footwear. This is particularly important in the ward toilet, or on the bedside commode. Elderly people, particularly, become cold very quickly, and the nurse should ensure that patients are not left exposed for more than the minimum time required for toileting.

The temperature of ward areas and toilet areas should remain at an environmentally comfortable level.

Mobilising

The choice of toilet arrangements for a particular patient, and the decision to use mechanical aids may depend on the patients' individually assessed activity of mobilising. The choice of arrangements should be discussed and accepted by the patient.

Expressing sexuality

When a patient needs help with toilet requirements it is an invasion of his privacy. The nurse may have to touch areas of the body which would normally be socially unacceptable, and may cause embarrassment to the patient. The nurse's attitude and good communication skills will help to alleviate some of the embarrassment felt by the patient although he may never be completely happy about this nursing practice.

Sleeping

Toilet facilities should be offered immediately prior to settling the patient for the night, so that maximum comfort is achieved. The nurse should also assure the patient that if he needs help for toileting during the night it will be readily available, ensuring that his bell or other means of communication is at hand.

Suggested reading
Barron A 1990 The right to personal space. Nursing Times 86(27) July 4: 28–33
Rooney V 1987 Toileting charts. Nursing 3(22) October: 827–830
Roper N, Logan W, Tierney A 1990 The elements of nursing, 3rd edn. Churchill
    Livingstone, Edinburgh, pp 177–201
Swaffield J 1988 Motivating for continence. Nursing Times 84(43) October 26: 56, 59
Tierney A (ed) 1986 Clinical nursing practice. Recent advances in nursing 14. Churchill
    Livingstone, Edinburgh, pp 47–75
Walsh M, Ford P 1989 Nursing rituals, research and rational actions. Heinemann
    Nursing, Oxford pp 68–69
Wilson M 1987 Elimination. Nursing 3(16) April: 612–615

Specimen Collection

There are three parts to this section:

1 Collection of a midstream specimen of urine
2 Collection of a catheter specimen of urine
3 Collection of a specimen of faeces

The concluding subsection, 'Relevance to the activities of living', refers to the three practices collectively.

Objectives

By the end of this section you should know how to:

- prepare the patient for all three nursing practices
- collect and prepare the equipment
- carry out collection of a midstream specimen of urine, a catheter specimen of urine and a specimen of faeces

Related information

Review of health authority policy on the collection and transportation of specimens.

Revision of urine testing (see p. 204).

1 COLLECTION OF A MIDSTREAM SPECIMEN OF URINE

Some indications for collection of a midstream specimen of urine

This is the collection of a specimen of urine for microbiological analysis, which has not been contaminated with microorganisms from outside the urinary system:

- to aid in the diagnosis of disease
- to assist in identifying the appropriate drug therapy
- to monitor the effect of treatment of disease

Equipment

Bedpan/urinal or toilet pan
Warm saline solution or soap and water for cleansing of the genitalia
Sterile gallipot
Sterile cotton wool balls
Sterile disposable gloves
Sterile receiver
Sterile specimen container appropriately labelled with a completed laboratory form and plastic specimen bag for transportation
Tray for equipment
Receptacle for soiled disposables
Disposable gloves

Guidelines for this nursing practice

- explain the nursing practice to the patient and gain his consent and cooperation
- collect and prepare the equipment required
- ensure the patient's privacy
- observe the patient throughout this activity

- position the bedpan/urinal or help the patient to the toilet
- help the patient into a comfortable position
- wash the hands
- open and arrange the equipment
- apply sterile gloves

Female patient

- cleanse the labia and urethral meatus using one swab once only, swabbing from front to back to reduce contamination from the anal region

- separate the labia and maintain this position until the specimen is collected in order to reduce contamination of the urine specimen

Male patient

- retract the foreskin, cleanse the glans penis and urethral meatus

- maintain the position of the retracted foreskin until the specimen is collected in order to reduce contamination of the urine specimen, then replace the foreskin

Both sexes

- ask the patient to begin micturition then stop. This will clear the distal urethra of contaminants
- place the sterile receiver in position
- ask the patient to micturate again then stop
- remove receiver and allow the patient to finish micturition
- pour the specimen into the sterile container
- ensure that the patient is left feeling as comfortable as possible

- dispose of the equipment safely
- place the specimen container into a specimen bag
- dispatch the labelled specimen to the laboratory immediately with the completed laboratory form
- document the nursing practice appropriately, monitor after-effects and report abnormal findings immediately

2   COLLECTION OF A CATHETER SPECIMEN OF URINE

Some indications for collection of a catheter specimen of urine

This is the collection of a specimen of urine for microbiological analysis, from a patient who has a retained catheter:

- to aid in the diagnosis of disease
- to assist in identifying the appropriate drug therapy
- to monitor the effect of treatment of disease

Equipment

Alcohol-saturated sterile swab, e.g. Mediswab
Sterile syringe and needle
Catheter clamp
Sterile specimen container appropriately labelled with a completed laboratory form and plastic specimen bag for transportation
Tray for equipment
Receptacle for soiled disposables
Disposable gloves

Guidelines for this nursing practice

- explain the nursing practice to the patient and gain his consent and cooperation
- collect and prepare the equipment required
- ensure the patient's privacy
- observe the patient throughout this activity
- clamp the drainage bag tubing below the rubber self-sealing sleeve for approximately 15 minutes to allow urine to accumulate
- wash the hands
- apply gloves
- cleanse the rubber sleeve with the alcohol-saturated swab
- insert the assembled needle and syringe at a 45° angle into the rubber sleeve
- withdraw the urine specimen (Fig. 5.1)

- remove the needle and syringe and wipe the rubber sleeve with the alcohol-saturated swab
- introduce the collected specimen of urine into the sterile container
- remove the clamp to re-establish the flow of urine
- ensure the patient is left feeling as comfortable as possible
- dispose of the equipment safely
- place the specimen container into the specimen bag
- dispatch the labelled specimen to the laboratory immediately with the completed laboratory form
- document the nursing practice appropriately, monitor after-effects and report abnormal findings immediately

3   COLLECTION OF A SPECIMEN OF FAECES

Some indications for collection of a specimen of faeces

- to aid in the diagnosis of disease

Equipment

Bedpan
Sterile spatula
Sterile specimen container appropriately labelled with a completed laboratory form and a plastic specimen bag for transportation
Tray for equipment
Receptacle for soiled disposables

Guidelines for this nursing practice

- explain the nursing practice to the patient and gain his consent and cooperation

- collect and prepare the equipment

- ensure the patient's privacy

- ask the patient to defaecate into the bedpan without urinating and thus contaminating the faecal matter. A male patient will require a urinal

- remove the bedpan and ensure the patient is left feeling as comfortable as possible

- wash the hands

- observe the colour, amount and consistency of the faeces

- using the sterile spatula place a specimen of faeces into the sterile container

- dispose of the equipment safely

- place the specimen container into the specimen bag

- dispatch the labelled specimen to the laboratory immediately with the completed laboratory form

- document the nursing practice appropriately, monitor after-effects and report abnormal findings immediately

Figure 5.1
Collecting a specimen of urine when a catheter is in position

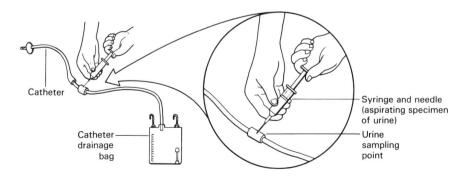

Catheter

Catheter drainage bag

Syringe and needle (aspirating specimen of urine)

Urine sampling point

Specimen Collection

Relevance to the activities of living

Maintaining a safe environment

Thorough cleansing of the patient's genitalia must be carried out prior to the collection of the specimen to reduce the number of contaminants from outside the urinary and intestinal systems. Antiseptics should not be used for cleansing as this would alter the number of pathogenic microorganisms, leading to inaccurate laboratory results.

Human tissue and body fluids such as urine and faeces can act as a health hazard to the staff handling the specimen, therefore gloves can be worn during collection to prevent staff contamination. The specimen container should only be half to a third full and checked for lid security to reduce the problem of leakage. The use of a plastic specimen container bag for transportation will help to prevent any health hazard to the staff, should accidental breakage of the specimen container occur. When a patient requires source isolation all precautions prior to, during and following specimen collection must be maintained.

Once collected, the specimen should be dispatched immediately to the laboratory. Should there be a delay the specimen must be stored at 4°C in a special refrigerator to reduce further growth of the pathogenic microorganisms. Urine specimen containers which contain boric acid crystals can be used when a delay in the dispatch of the specimen is anticipated, as boric acid acts as a urine preservative.

A catheter specimen of urine should not be collected by disconnecting the drainage bag from the catheter or by taking the specimen from the outlet tap of the urine drainage bag. The former method has the potential of allowing pathogenic microorganisms to have access to the urinary system; the latter will not give a specimen of urine which will contain the 'true' pathogenic microorganisms present in the urinary system. Care has to be taken during the collection of a cathether specimen of urine to prevent the accidental stabbing of the nurse's finger by advancing the needle too far and going through the drainage tubing.

Communicating

The patient should be given an easily understood explanation as to how and why the specimen collection is required. The laboratory results should be conveyed to the patient as soon as possible. Both of these actions will reduce patient anxiety.

A patient who has a urinary tract infection, or has just had surgery to the urinary system, may suffer urinary muscle spasm and/or pain. The medical practitioner may prescribe appropriate analgesics and antispasmodics which can be of great benefit to the patient.

Eating and drinking

A patient who is suspected of having a bacterial or viral infection of the urinary or intestinal systems may suffer from thirst, nausea, vomiting and/or loss of appetite. The nurse will require to initiate the appropriate nursing intervention to help the patient.

Eliminating

Frequent micturition should be encouraged when a urinary infection is suspected. This will reduce the time the pathogenic microorganisms have for multiplication within the patient's urinary system.

When collecting a specimen, the urine and/or faeces should be observed for colour, amount, consistency and any obvious abnormality.

A faecal specimen may be requested for bacterial or viral studies, but can be requested for biochemical analysis such as testing for the presence of faecal occult blood. This test is now carried out at ward level by a nurse using a commercial biochemical testing kit such as Haemocult. The nurse should acquaint herself with the manufacturer's recommendations for use.

A stool chart may be initiated when a patient has a suspected intestinal infection. This records the frequency, colour, consistency and amount of faecal matter passed by the patient. The stool chart can be used as an aid to diagnosis and assists in the assessment of the effect of treatment.

Sleeping

A patient with a suspected infection of the urinary or intestinal systems may suffer from an increase/urgency of micturition and defaecation, which may interrupt sleeping. The nurse should assist the patient with this problem by initiating the appropriate nursing intervention.

Suggested reading   Brunner L, Suddarth D 1988 Textbook of medical–surgical nursing. J. B. Lippincott, Philadelphia, pp 747–748, 1000–1002

Glenister H 1983 Diagnosis of the patient and specimen collection. Nursing 2(19) November, Supplement: 6

Long B, Phipps W 1985 Essentials of medical–surgical nursing – a nursing process approach. C.V. Mosby, St Louis, pp 947–949

Pearson F 1980 Collection of stool specimens. Nursing 1(17) September: 756–757

Roper N, Logan W, Tierney A 1990 The elements of nursing, 3rd edn. Churchill Livingstone, Edinburgh, pp 183–187

Silvester G 1984 Investigation of the gastrointestinal tract. Nursing 2(30) October: 896–897

Wallis M 1984 The collection and testing of urine. Nursing 2(29) September: 853–854

Testing Urine

Objectives

By the end of this section you should know how to:

- prepare the patient for this nursing practice
- collect the equipment required
- carry out testing of urine

Related information

Revision of the anatomy and physiology of the urinary system with special reference to the formation of urine

Revision of the manufacturer's instructions for the chemical reagents to be used.

Some indications for testing urine

Testing urine is the assessment of the constituents of urine by observational, biochemical and mechanical means:

- to aid in the diagnosis of disease
- to assist in the monitoring of disease and treatment
- to assist in the assessment of the health of an individual
- to exclude pathology

Equipment

Container for urine sample
Bottle of reagent strips and/or reagent tablets
Test tube if appropriate and test tube rack
Pipette
Jug for volume measurement
Bedpan or urinal
Watch with seconds hand
Trolley or tray for equipment
Receptacle for soiled disposables
Disposable gloves

Guidelines for this nursing practice

- explain the nursing practice to the patient and obtain his consent and cooperation

- instruct or assist the patient to collect urine in the clean container the next time he empties his bladder

- collect and prepare the equipment

- wash the hands

- apply gloves

- measure the volume of urine if the patient has a fluid balance chart

- observe and note any sediment present in the urine

- observe and note the colour of the urine

- check the date of expiry on the container of reagent strips and/or reagent tablets

Reagent strips

- remove a reagent strip, being careful not to touch the test squares on the strip as this could give a false reading

- immerse the reagent strip fully in the urine: note the time

- read the reagent strip after the recommended time has elapsed

- note the results

Reagent tablet

- remove a reagent tablet from the bottle, placing it on a clean dry surface

- prepare the urine sample as recommended by the manufacturer

- utilise the reagent tablet as instructed by the manufacturer

- note the result of the test after the recommended time

Reagent strip and tablet

- dispose of the equipment safely

- document the nursing practice appropriately and report abnormal findings immediately

Relevance to the activities of living

Maintaining a safe environment

Although testing urine does not require aseptic technique, all equipment should be clean or disposable and all precautions be taken to prevent cross-infection. The nurse should wash her hands before commencing, and on completion of, the nursing practice.

All chemical reagents should be stored in a locked cupboard or drawer to comply with health and safety at work regulations.

When a patient is asked to collect a specimen of urine for routine testing, the container to be used must be clean and dry. It is essential that the container is free from contaminating substances as this may lead to inaccurate results.

Once the urine sample has been obtained it should be tested immediately. Urine constituents can alter when left exposed to the environment, which may predispose to inaccurate results.

The manufacturer's instructions for care and storage should be followed precisely. These chemical reagents are liable to degradation over a period of time or when storage conditions are not adequate. It is essential that the lid of the container is replaced securely following removal of a reagent strip or tablet, as they are particularly sensitive to changes in temperature and humidity. The chemical reagents should be handled carefully. Touching of the test square or tablet could introduce contaminants which may alter the results obtained. When using a reagent strip, hold the strip horizontally or place over the urine container. This will prevent any excess urine dripping onto the nurse's hand which could be a health hazard to the member of staff. Holding the strip horizontally will also prevent mixing of the urine between the test squares which may lead to inaccurate results.

It is important that the reagent strip or tablet test is read at the time specified by the manufacturer. Reading the test too late or too soon would give inaccurate results.

Communicating

The patient will require a full and easily understood explanation as to why the urine specimen is required and how to collect the specimen.

The nurse should familiarise herself with any medications the patient may be taking, as certain drugs can affect the test.

Eliminating

Fresh urine from a healthy individual should not have an offensive odour, but decomposing urine will smell like ammonia. A patient whose urine is found to have a 'sweet smell' may be investigated further for diabetes mellitus. Urine smelling of fish can be an indication of infection of the urinary system.

The normal colour of urine will range from pale straw to dark amber and the colour of a patient's urine will vary according to the amount of fluid taken into the body. The type and amount of urine constituents will also affect the colour of urine, e.g. dark coloured urine can be an indication of dehydration or the presence of bile pigments – a manifestation of liver or biliary tract disease.

Certain drugs will alter the colour of a patient's urine.

Haematuria is the term used to describe blood in the urine. This can vary from microscopic haematuria, i.e. detected only by testing, through to frank haematuria, i.e. an obvious red coloration.

Glycosuria is the term used when there is sugar in the urine, and it is suggestive of diabetes mellitus.

Proteinuria is the term used when there is protein in the urine, which can be a manifestation of acute or chronic renal disease.

When the body metabolises fat, ketones are one of the products of this metabolism. Ketones are acidotic, and if excessive metabolism of fat persists, a state of metabolic acidosis develops which if untreated can lead to coma and death. At a certain stage of acidosis, the ketones are excreted by the urinary system, and when identified in urine may be indicative of excessive fasting or uncontrolled or poorly controlled diabetes mellitus.

Specific gravity is a measure of the concentration of the substances dissolved in the urine and the normal range is 1.005–1.025. A single measurement of the specific gravity of urine will give little information, as the specific gravity varies depending on the state of hydration of the body. Urine which continually measures a low specific gravity is a manifestation of renal damage or diabetes insipidus. The pH of a urine sample is an indicator of kidney function in maintaining the acid–base balance within the body.

Expressing sexuality

Micturition is an activity associated with privacy and collecting a specimen of urine is usually an unfamiliar experience for the patient, therefore providing privacy and giving an adequate explanation of the practice will be conducive to an uncomplicated collection of the specimen.

When asking a female patient for a urine specimen it is necessary to ask her if she is menstruating, as the menstrual flow may give a falsely positive urine blood result.

Suggested reading

Ames Division Aids to diagnosis – a short technical manual, 3rd edn. Bayer Diagnostics UK, Slough (available from Bayer Diagnostics UK Limited, Stoke Court, Stoke Poges, Slough SL2 4LY)

Bowker C (ed) 1986 Focus on urinalysis.
1. Anatomy and physiology of renal tract. Nursing Times Supplement 81(17) April 23: 1–6
2. Collection of urine samples. Nursing Times Supplement 81(20) May 14: 1–6
3. Urine testing. Nursing Times Supplement 81(23) June 4: 1–6
4. Case history – diabetes: urine tests for glucose and ketones. Nursing Times Supplement 81(26) June 25: 1–6
5. Proteinuria. Case history – liver function tests: differential diagnosis of jaundice: urine tests for bilirubin and urobilinogen. Nursing Times Supplement 81(29) July 16: 1–6
6. Regulation of water balance–specific gravity: urinary pH: urinary tract infection: haematuria. Nursing Times Supplement 81(32) August 6: 1–6

Roper N, Logan W, Tierney A 1990 The elements of nursing, 3rd edn. Churchill Livingstone, Edinburgh, pp 183–187

Royal College of Nursing 1990 Urinalysis – a critical analysis. (Video) Healthcare Productions Limited, London

Wallis M 1984 The collection and testing of urine. Nursing 2(29) September: 853–854

Urinary Catheterisation

There are four parts to this section:

1 **Catheterisation**
2 **Catheter care**
3 **Bladder irrigation**
4 **Bladder lavage**

The concluding subsection 'Relevance to the activities of living' refers to the four practices collectively.

Objectives

By the end of this section you should know how to:

- prepare the patient for these four nursing practices
- collect and prepare the equipment
- carry out catheterisation, catheter care, bladder irrigation and bladder lavage

Related information

Revision of the anatomy and physiology of the urinary system and external genitalia.

Revision of aseptic technique (see p. 26).

1   CATHETERISATION

Some indications for urethral catheterisation

Urethral catheterisation is the passing of a catheter through the urethral orifice to the bladder:

- to re-establish a flow of urine in urinary retention
- to provide a channel for drainage when micturition is impaired
- to maintain a dry environment in urinary incontinence when all other forms of nursing intervention have failed
- to empty the bladder preoperatively
- to allow monitoring of fluid balance in a seriously ill patient
- to facilitate bladder irrigation procedures

Equipment

Good light source, such as spotlight
Sterile gloves
Sterile catheterisation pack or dressings pack
Sterile water-based antiseptic for cleansing the genitalia
Sterile anaesthetic gel if required, or water-soluble lubricant
Sterile receiver
Sterile catheter of type and size required
Sterile closed drainage system if required
Hypoallergenic tape
Sterile specimen container appropriately labelled with a completed laboratory form and plastic specimen bag for transportation
Trolley for equipment
Receptacle for soiled disposables

Catheters

The reason for urinary catheterisation can dictate the type and size of catheter (Fig. 5.2) to be used, e.g.:
— Round-ended catheter can be used when a retained catheter is not required
— Foley double lumen self-retaining catheter can be used when a short-term retained catheter is required
— Foley triple lumen self-retaining catheter can be used when continuous bladder irrigation is required
— Tiemann catheter can be used when the urethral canal is narrowed, such as occurs when a male patient has an enlarged prostate gland: the shape of the catheter tip aids the passage of the catheter
— Whistle-tipped catheter can be used postoperatively to allow the passage of blood clots, particularly when bladder irrigation is not being utilised
— Silastic catheter can be used when a retained catheter is required for long-term use, as silastic is less irritant to the body tissue

Sizes:
— 14 FG is a suitable size of catheter for a female patient
— 14 FG–16 FG is a suitable size of catheter for a male patient

Larger-sized catheters may be used when the urine has an excess of sediment and/or blood

Catheters are manufactured in female and male catheter lengths

Figure 5.2
Catheterisation: examples of catheters (Key: 1 = channel for urine flow; 2 = channel for balloon inflation; 3 = channel for irrigating fluid flow)

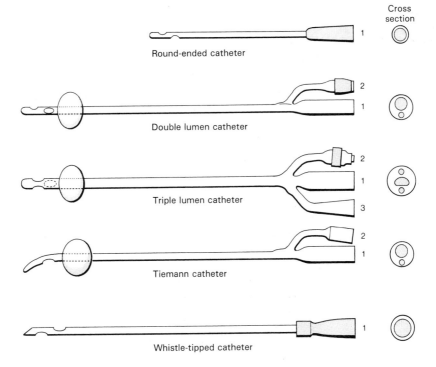

Cross section

Round-ended catheter

Double lumen catheter

Triple lumen catheter

Tiemann catheter

Whistle-tipped catheter

Urinary Catheterisation

Guidelines for this nursing practice

Female patient

- explain the nursing practice to the patient and obtain her consent and cooperation
- collect and prepare the equipment
- ensure the patient's privacy
- observe the patient throughout this activity
- prepare and help the patient into a supine position with knees bent, hips flexed, and feet resting on the bed approximately 0.7 m apart
- place an incontinence pad or similar waterproof sheet under the patient's buttocks

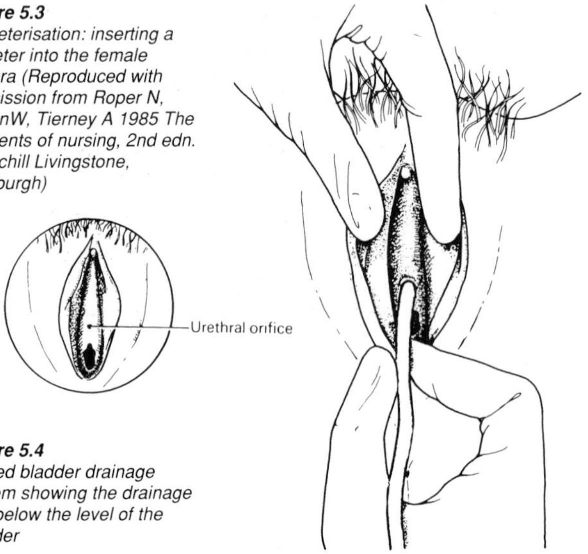

Figure 5.3
Catheterisation: inserting a catheter into the female urethra (Reproduced with permission from Roper N, LoganW, Tierney A 1985 The elements of nursing, 2nd edn. Churchill Livingstone, Edinburgh)

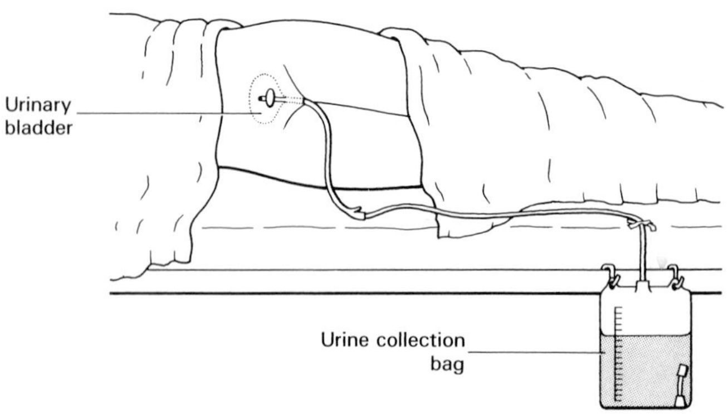

Urethral orifice

Figure 5.4
Closed bladder drainage system showing the drainage bag below the level of the bladder

Urinary bladder

Urine collection bag

- arrange the lighting
- wash the hands and put on the gloves
- open and arrange the equipment using an aseptic technique
- observe the patient throughout this activity
- cleanse the labia minora swabbing from above downwards to reduce the danger of cross-infection from the anal region
- using the non-dominant hand, separate the labia minora to reveal the urethral meatus until the completion of insertion of the catheter
- with the dominant hand cleanse the urethral meatus and position the sterile receiver
- insert the lubricated catheter into the urethra in an upward and backward direction avoiding contamination of the surface of the catheter until a flow of urine is established (Fig. 5.3)
- exert gentle pressure just above the level of the symphysis pubis to assist drainage from the bladder
- if it is not intended that the catheter should be left in situ, gently remove the catheter when the urine flow ceases
- if for retention, gently advance the catheter 4–5 cm and inflate the balloon according to the manufacturer's directions. Attach a closed drainage system (Fig. 5.4)
- anchor the catheter when appropriate by taping the catheter and drainage tubing to the thigh to reduce catheter movement within the bladder and urethra
- ensure that the patient is left feeling as comfortable as possible
- dispose of the equipment safely
- document the nursing practice appropriately, monitor after-effects and report abnormal findings immediately

Male patient

This is usually carried out by a medical practitioner or a male nurse.

- explain the nursing practice to the patient and obtain his consent and cooperation

- collect and prepare the equipment

- ensure the patient's privacy

- observe the patient throughout this activity

- prepare and help the patient into a supine position

- place an incontinence pad or similar waterproof sheet under the patient's buttocks and arrange the lighting

- wash the hands and put on the gloves

- open and arrange the equipment using an aseptic technique

- withdraw the patient's foreskin and maintain this with the non-dominant hand

- with the dominant hand cleanse the glans penis and urethral meatus

- insert the lignocaine gel and leave for 2 minutes to allow the local anaesthetic to act

- position the sterile receiver and with the non-dominant hand gently grasp the shaft of the penis raising it straight up and insert the lubricated catheter into the urethral meatus for approximately 20–25 cm, until a flow of urine is established (Fig. 5.5)

- continue as for the Guidelines in the female patient until the anchoring of the catheter

- replace the patient's foreskin over the glans penis, otherwise a paraphimosis may develop

- anchor the catheter by taping laterally to the thigh or abdomen

- ensure that the patient is left feeling as comfortable as possible

- dispose of the equipment safely

- document the nursing practice appropriately, monitor after-effects, and report abnormal findings immediately

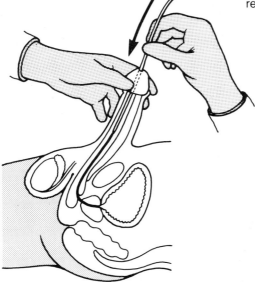

Figure 5.5
Catheterisation: inserting a catheter into the male urethra

2   CATHETER CARE

Some indications for catheter care

Catheter care is the cleansing of the exposed part of a catheter which may:

- help reduce the risk of ascending infection via the catheter to other parts of the urinary system

- remove any crusts or discharge from the catheter as they can harbour pathogenic microorganisms

Equipment

Sterile disposable gloves
Sterile swabs or cotton wool balls
Sterile gallipot
Sterile water-based antiseptic solution or normal saline
Sterile antiseptic cream
Tray for equipment
Receptacle for soiled disposables

Guidelines for this nursing practice

- explain the nursing practice to the patient and obtain his consent and cooperation

- collect and prepare the equipment

- ensure the patient's privacy

- observe the patient throughout this activity

- help the patient into a suitable position

- wash the hands and arrange the equipment

- gently cleanse the external urethral meatus, swabbing from above downwards in the female patient to reduce the risk of cross-infection

- in a male patient retract the foreskin before cleansing and replace following completion of this nursing practice

- gently swab the shaft of the catheter to remove any discharge swabbing away from the urethral orifice

- apply antiseptic cream to the catheter–meatal junction

- ensure that the patient is left feeling as comfortable as possible

- dispose of the equipment safely

- document the nursing practice appropriately, monitor after-effects and report abnormal findings immediately

3 BLADDER IRRIGATION

Some indications for bladder irrigation

Bladder irrigation is the continuous washing out of the bladder using sterile fluid.

Continuous bladder irrigation can be carried out through a three-way urethral catheter or through suprapubic and urethral catheters:

- to prevent blood clot formation following surgery to the urinary tract
- to clear an obstructed catheter
- to aid removal of blood clots and/or sediment in the bladder

Equipment

Sterile dressings pack
Sterile water-based antiseptic lotion
Sterile irrigating solution at 37.8°C, e.g. normal saline, chlorhexidine 0.02% in water
Sterile irrigation set
Sterile drainage bag with outlet tap
Catheter clamp
Trolley for equipment
Receptacle for soiled disposables

Guidelines for this nursing practice

- explain the nursing practice to the patient and gain his consent and cooperation
- collect and prepare the equipment
- ensure the patient's privacy
- observe the patient throughout this activity
- help the patient into a comfortable position
- wash the hands
- open the dressings pack and arrange equipment
- clamp the urethral catheter
- cleanse the inlet arm of the catheter with the antiseptic solution
- insert the irrigation set connector into the inlet arm of the catheter
- attach the urine drainage bag if a drainage bag is not already in use
- remove the catheter clamp
- allow the accumulated urine to drain and empty the drainage bag
- open the valve on the irrigation set and regulate to the prescribed rate
- ensure that the patient is left feeling as comfortable as possible
- dispose of the equipment safely
- document the nursing practice, monitor after-effects and report abnormal findings immediately

4   BLADDER LAVAGE

Some indications for bladder lavage

Bladder lavage is the intermittent washing out of the bladder using sterile fluid:

- to aid removal of sediment and/or blood clots
- to clear an obstructed catheter
- to allow administration of medicine into the bladder

Equipment

Sterile disposable gloves
Sterile dressings pack
Sterile water-based antiseptic solution
Sterile lavage fluid at 37.8°C, e.g. normal saline
Sterile 50 ml bladder syringe
2 sterile receivers
Sterile drainage bag
Catheter clamp
Large clean receiver for returned lavage fluid
Trolley for equipment
Receptacle for soiled disposables

Guidelines for this nursing practice

- explain the nursing practice to the patient and gain his consent and cooperation
- collect and prepare the equipment required
- ensure the patient's privacy
- observe the patient throughout this activity
- help the patient into a comfortable position
- wash the hands
- open the dressings pack and arrange equipment
- clamp the urethral catheter, disconnect the drainage bag and discard
- cleanse the end of the catheter with the antiseptic solution using the dressing forceps or a gloved hand
- place one sterile receiver under the catheter
- charge the bladder syringe with the lavage solution which has been poured into the second receiver
- release the clamp on the catheter
- introduce all the solution slowly into the bladder and then allow this fluid to flow into the sterile receiver
- repeat until the prescribed volume of fluid has been used
- attach the sterile drainage bag
- ensure that the patient is left feeling as comfortable as possible
- dispose of the equipment safely
- compare the volume of fluid injected with the fluid returned; discrepancies should be documented
- document the nursing practice appropriately, monitor after-effects and report abnormal findings immediately

Relevance to the activities of living

Maintaining a safe environment

Introducing a catheter into the bladder has the potential to allow pathogenic microorganisms to enter a sterile environment in a healthy individual and therefore the nurse must be vigilant in maintaining aseptic technique throughout the practice. Anchoring of the catheter reduces the potential problem of trauma to the internal and external urethral sphincters and bladder tissue, and a self-retaining catheter with a small balloon may help reduce the trauma to the bladder epithelium.

The maintenance of a closed drainage system and the use of appropriate infection control measures when emptying a drainage bag will help reduce the potential problem of ascending infection to the urinary system (Fig. 5.6). Instillation of antiseptic solution through the outlet tap of the drainage bag can discourage the growth of pathogens: one of the main entry points for infection is the catheter–meatal junction. The benefit of catheter care in reducing the risk of ascending infection remains unclear, therefore the nurse should be guided by local policy.

During bladder lavage, the connection between the catheter and drainage bag is broken and this creates the potential problem of introducing pathogens to the urinary tract. Because of this danger, some health agencies do not advocate bladder lavage.

To prevent blockage by blood clots and/or sediment, a catheter may require regular 'milking' of the tubing. Maintaining a clear flow of urine helps to prevent stagnation of urine and therefore prevents infection of the bladder and urinary tract.

Communicating

The patient must be given an easily understood explanation about the reason for the commencement of any of the nursing practices listed. If these practices are to be used as part of a patient's postoperative care, the explanation should be given preoperatively, and this will help to reduce patient anxiety.

The patient's anxiety must be further reduced by explaining the reason for the appearance and colour of the drainage fluid during a bladder irrigation or lavage.

The patient may experience pain during a bladder irrigation due to the irrigation of the raw areas of the bladder by the irrigating solution. Analgesia should be given as prescribed by the medical practitioner.

Eliminating

Drainage of urine via a catheter is a deviation from the normal method of micturition but does not interfere with normal defaecation.

Before cleansing of the urethra the nurse should look for any urethral discharge. Any resistance felt during the passage of the catheter, and any bleeding from the urethra following insertion of the catheter, should be noted.

The nurse should note and record the quantity of urine drained from the patient's bladder. If the catheter has been inserted to re-establish urine flow in urinary retention, only 500 ml of urine should be drained in the first hour. The catheter should then be clamped and 200–300 ml of urine be drained every hour until the patient's bladder is empty. This will help to prevent loss of bladder muscle tone following an acute retention of urine.

Figure 5.6
Points at which pathogens can enter a closed urinary drainage system:
1 the urethral orifice
2 connection of catheter and drainage tube
3 where sample of urine is taken
4 connection of drainage tube and collecting bag
5 drainage bag outlet
(Reproduced with permission from Roper N, Logan W, Tierney A 1985 The elements of nursing, 2nd edn. Churchill Livingstone, Edinburgh)

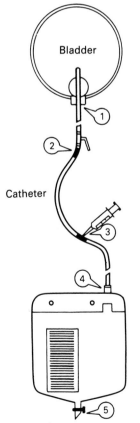

Bladder

Catheter

Relevance to the
activities of living
continued

The colour of the urine should be noted. Pale pink to red through to brown is suggestive of blood in the urine – haematuria. Blood or sediment in the urine is suggestive of a malfunction of the renal or urinary systems due to disease or trauma, and should therefore be noted. It should be remembered that certain medicines such as rifampicin (an anti-tuberculosis medication) can colour the urine reddish-brown and is not a cause for alarm.

Following the commencement of a bladder irrigation the rate of infusion of the irrigating solution will usually be dependent on the appearance of the fluid returned into the urine drainage bag. Following surgery such as a prostatectomy, the patient may require an irrigating volume of 5–10 l in the first 12 hours, but this volume of fluid can usually be reduced to 3–5 l during the following 12–18 hour period. The amount and appearance of the fluid removed from the drainage bag should be recorded and, following surgery, fluid which appears to be rose in colour indicates an adequate irrigation rate. The patient's urinary output is calculated by subtracting the amount of drained fluid from the volume of infused irrigating solution. Any resistance or inability to introduce the irrigating or lavage fluid should be reported and documented appropriately.

Eating and drinking

Assistance should be given to the patient to increase his oral fluid intake. This will promote an increase in the volume of fluid passing through the urinary system and bladder which will help to prevent a urinary tract infection developing due to urinary stagnation. An accurate fluid balance chart must be maintained at all times. Should the patient have both an intravenous infusion and a bladder irrigation system in position, care must be taken not to confuse the urinary irrigation set and solution, with the intravenous giving set and fluid.

Personal cleansing and dressing

When a catheter is retained over a long period, it is important to ensure that perineal hygiene is maintained and this may involve some education of the patient. He should be advised to wear loose underwear which is less likely to compress the catheter tubing.

Mobilising

If a catheter is retained, it along with the drainage tubing may impede mobilising. Interference may be reduced by using leg drainage bags, which can be easily anchored to the patient's leg.

Expressing sexuality

Introduction of a catheter could be perceived by the patient as an 'assault' on body image. Adequate provision of privacy during catheterisation and catheter care is conducive to reducing the patient's anxiety and embarrassment, and use of a ward treatment room is preferable to a screened bed in an open ward.

The appearance of a retained catheter and urine drainage bag can cause a patient a great deal of embarrassment and anxiety. The discreet placement of the urine drainage bag out of the obvious vision of visitors and other patients will be greatly appreciated by the embarrassed patient and leg drainage bags are less visible and more comfortable.

When a patient with an indwelling catheter is being discharged home, advice should be given to the patient and the partner about sexual activity.

Sleeping

A retained catheter may interfere with a patient's usual sleep pattern. As the patient moves during sleep the catheter and/or tubing could become trapped causing the patient to awaken due to the discomfort caused by tension on the catheter; this possibility should be discussed with the patient, in order to reduce alarm should it occur.

Suggested reading

Britton P, Wright E 1990 Catheters: making an informed choice. Professional Nurse 5(4) January: 194–198

Gilbert V, Gobbi M 1989 Making sense of bladder irrigation. Nursing Times 85(16) April 19: 40–42

Glenister H 1990 Investigating infection acquired in hospitals. Nursing Times 86(49) December 5: 46–48

Hamilton B 1985 Have catheter, will travel. Nursing Times Community Outlook 81(41) October 9: 16–17

Kennedy A, Brocklehurst J, Lye M 1983 Factors relating to the problems of long term catheterisation. Journal of Advanced Nursing 8(3) May: 207–212

Lowthian P 1989 Preventing trauma. Nursing Times 85(21) May 24: 73–75

O'Neil G 1986 A drain on resources (new technique for catheterisation). Nursing Times 82(38) September 17: 89–90

Pick D 1990 Standards of excellence (a standard for catheter care). Nursing 4(2) December 6: 17–18

Pillmoor M 1988 Urinary tract infection – a nursing perspective. Surgical Nurse 1(6) December: 21–25

Rees-Williams C, Meyrick M, Jones M 1988 Making sense of urinary catheters. Nursing Times 84(40) October 5: 46–47

Roe B 1990 Do we need to clamp catheters? Nursing Times 86(43) October 24: 66–67

Roe B 1990 Catheter prescribing and the use of antimicrobials. Nursing Times 86(14) December 5: 46–48

Roe B, Chapman R, Crow R 1986 A study of the procedures for catheter care recommended by District Health Authorities and Schools of Nursing. Nursing Practice Research Unit, University of Surrey, Guildford

Roper N, Logan W, Tierney A 1990 The elements of nursing, 3rd edn. Churchill Livingstone, Edinburgh, ch 10

Walsh M, Ford P 1989 Nursing rituals – research and rational actions. Heinemann Nursing, London: pp 19–21

Winder A 1990 Intermittent self-catheterisation. Nursing Times 86(43) October 24: 63–64

Rectal Examination

Objectives

By the end of this section you should know how to:

- prepare the patient for this procedure
- collect and prepare the equipment
- assist the medical practitioner as requested

Related information

Revision of the anatomy and physiology of the sigmoid colon, rectum and anus.

Some indications for rectal examination

Rectal examination is used as a diagnostic aid when there is:

- rectal bleeding
- severe constipation
- pain in the anal or rectal area
- suspected enlarged prostate gland
- suspected rectocele

Outline of the procedure

The medical practitioner will put a disposable glove on his dominant hand and apply some lubricant to his fingertips. He will then insert one or two fingers into the patient's rectum and perform the examination. On completing the examination he will remove the glove by turning it inside out as he takes it off. He may insert a lubricated rectal speculum and, using the light source, carry out a visual examination.

Equipment

Tray
Disposable gloves
Sterile rectal speculum (Fig. 5.7)
Water-soluble lubricant
Protective covering for the bed
Receptacle for soiled disposables
Swabs
Light source

Figure 5.7
Rectal speculum

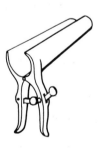

Guidelines for this nursing practice

- help explain the procedure to the patient and gain his consent and cooperation
- collect and prepare the equipment
- assist the patient into the position requested by the medical practitioner, ensuring privacy
- observe the patient throughout this activity
- assist the medical practitioner as requested
- ensure the patient is left feeling as comfortable as possible
- dispose of the equipment safely
- document the examination in the patient's records, monitor after-effects and report abnormal findings immediately

Relevance to the activities of living

Maintaining a safe environment

The nurse and medical practitioner should wash their hands before commencing and on completion of the procedure.

Communicating

This can be a painful and embarrassing procedure for the patient so a careful explanation of the necessity for this examination should be given.

Breathing

It should be explained to the patient that he can help himself relax while the examination is taking place by breathing in and out slowly and deeply.

Eliminating

An empty rectum facilitates the examination but when there is rectal bleeding it is not advisable to administer suppositories or an enema.

Personal cleansing and dressing

Always ensure that the patient's anal area is clean and dry after this examination.

Expressing sexuality

This procedure can be embarrassing for the patient, so the nurse must ensure that there is maximum privacy while the examination is being conducted.

Suggested reading

Roberts A 1987 Systems of life, No. 147. Senior systems 12 – rectal bleeding. Nursing Times 83(11) March 18: 47–50
Roper N, Logan W, Tierney A 1990 The elements of nursing, 3rd edn. Churchill Livingstone, Edinburgh pp 198–199

Rectal Suppositories

Objectives

By the end of this section you should know how to:

- prepare the patient for this nursing practice
- collect and prepare the equipment
- administer rectal suppositories
- describe some of the types of suppositories and their function

Related information

Revision of the anatomy and physiology of the colon, rectum and anus.

Revision of medicine administration particularly checking the medication against the prescription (see p. 12).

(see p. 12)

Some indications for administering rectal suppositories

A suppository is a cone or cylinder of a medicinal substance which can be introduced into the rectum and will eventually dissolve. It is used:

- to relieve constipation
- to evacuate the bowel prior to surgery or certain investigations
- to administer medication, e.g. antibiotics, bronchodilators, analgesics

Equipment

Tray
Disposable gloves
Medical wipes
Water-soluble lubricant
Protective covering
Receptacle for soiled disposables
Prescribed suppository

Suppositories are of value in evacuating the rectum. Glycerine suppositories lubricate dry, hard stools and have a mild stimulant effect on the rectum. Other suppositories with a stimulant effect are Beogex and Bisacodyl.

Medication is well absorbed through the rectal mucosa. For many years, it has been a common way to administer medication in Europe, but it is only recently that it has become an acceptable route of administration to patients in the UK.

Guidelines for this nursing practice

- explain the nursing practice to the patient and gain his consent and cooperation
- ensure the patient's privacy and assist him into the left lateral position with his buttocks near the edge of the bed
- observe the patient throughout this activity
- place the protective covering under the patient's buttocks
- check with the prescription sheet and with a qualified member of staff that the suppository is the correct one and is being administered to the correct patient, if it is a means of administering a medication
- lubricate the end of the suppository
- put on the disposable gloves
- part the patient's buttocks with the non-dominant hand
- with the dominant hand insert the suppository into the rectum in an upward and slightly backward direction to follow the natural line of the rectum
- push the suppository in gently as far as possible with the middle finger
- withdraw the gloved finger
- wipe the patient's anal area with a medical wipe
- remove the protective covering
- remove the gloves
- provide a bedpan or commode when this is required
- ensure the patient is left feeling as comfortable as possible
- dispose of the equipment safely
- document this nursing practice appropriately, monitor after-effects and report any abnormal findings

Relevance to the activities of living

Communicating

It is important to explain clearly to the patient the reason for and method of action of the suppository.

Eliminating

If the suppository is being given to evacuate the rectum, the patient must have ready access to a bedpan, commode or toilet, and any necessary assistance should be given.

Expressing sexuality

Many patients find the administration of suppositories embarrassing so an adequate explanation should be given and maximum privacy must be provided.

Suggested reading

Boore J, Champion R, Ferguson M (eds) 1987 Nursing the physically ill adult. Churchill Livingstone, Edinburgh, ch 25
Ractoo S, Baumber C 1983 Testing times.Nursing Mirror 156(24) June 15: 26–27
Roper N, Logan W, Tierney A 1990 The elements of nursing, 3rd edn. Churchill Livingstone, Edinburgh, pp 185–187
Shreeve C 1985 Bowel habits in the elderly. Nursing Mirror 160(19) May 8: 20–21
Thomas M 1987 More fibre makes sense. Nursing Times 83(3) January 21: 39

Enemas

Objectives

By the end of this section you should know how to:

- prepare the patient for this nursing practice
- collect and prepare the equipment
- administer an enema
- describe the various enema preparations and their modes of action

Related information

Revision of the anatomy and physiology of the colon, rectum and anus.

Revision of drug administration, particularly checking the drug with the prescription (see p. 12).

Some indications for administering an enema

An enema is the introduction of liquid into the rectum by means of a tube. It is used:

- to relieve constipation
- to evacuate the bowel prior to surgery or investigations
- to administer medication

Equipment

Tray
Prescribed enema
Protective covering for the bed
Water-soluble lubricant
Disposable gloves
Commode or bedpan if required
Receptacle for soiled disposables

Types of enema (Fig. 5.8)

There are three main kinds:

- enemas containing medication, which should be retained as long as possible and should be inserted very slowly over half an hour
- stimulant enemas which are usually returned, with faecal matter and flatus, within a few minutes; a solution containing phosphates or sodium citrate is commonly used
- enemas which soften and lubricate faeces and should be retained for a specified time; they usually contain arachis or olive oil

At one time, a solution containing green soap was prescribed as an evacuant enema but it has been demonstrated that it can severely damage the mucosa of the bowel, and is no longer in use.

Guidelines for this nursing practice

- explain the nursing practice to the patient and gain his consent and cooperation
- assemble and prepare the equipment
- ensure the patient's privacy and help the patient into the left lateral position
- observe the patient throughout this activity
- place the protective covering under the patient's buttocks
- put on disposable gloves
- lubricate the end of the enema tube
- squeeze a small amount of fluid down the tube to expel the air
- insert the tube into the rectum in an upward and slightly backward direction for about 7.5 cm

- administer the solution gently and slowly
- remove the tube when the prescribed amount has been administered
- dry the anal area
- remove the protective covering
- provide a bedpan or commode when this is required
- ensure that the patient is left feeling as comfortable as possible
- dispose of the equipment safely
- document this nursing practice appropriately, monitor after-effects and report any abnormal findings immediately

Figure 5.8
Examples of disposable enemas

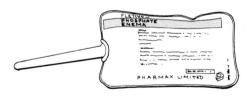

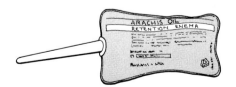

Enemas

Relevance to the activities of living

Maintaining a safe environment

Although this does not require aseptic technique, all the equipment used should be clean or disposable and the nurse should wash her hands before and on completion of the practice.

Care should be taken to avoid damaging the rectal mucosa when inserting the tube of the enema into the rectum. If the tube meets with resistance it should be withdrawn slightly and no force used.

Communicating

It is important to explain clearly to the patient the reason for the enema being prescribed so that he knows whether it has to be retained for a time or returned quickly.

Eating and drinking

If the enema is being administered to relieve constipation, advice should be given on how to help avoid this problem in the future. An increased intake of dietary fibre and fluids may be of benefit.

Eliminating

Ensure that the patient has ready access to a bedpan, commode or toilet, and that assistance is given where necessary.

Mobilising

Research has shown that bedfast or immobile patients have a greater tendency to suffer from constipation.

Expressing sexuality

This can be an embarrassing and distasteful practice for the patient, so maximum privacy must be given, plus a clear explanation of the necessity for the practice.

Suggested reading   Brooks S 1984 Disturbances of bowel function. Nursing 2(30) October: 870–876
Duffin H, Castleden C, Chaudhry A 1981 Are enemas necessary? Nursing Times 77(45) November 4: 1940–1941
Hamilton H (ed) 1985 Nurse's reference library – procedures. Springhouse Corporation, Pennsylvania, pp 575–580
Roper N, Logan W, Tierney A 1990 The elements of nursing, 3rd edn. Churchill Livingstone, Edinburgh, pp 185–187
Sadler C 1989 Elderly people with constipation. Nursing Times 3(44): 33
Shreeve C 1985 Bowel habits in the elderly. Nursing Mirror 160(19) May 8: 20–21
Wright L 1974 Bowel function in hospital patients. Royal College of Nursing, London

Bowel Washout

Objectives

By the end of this section you should know how to:

- prepare the patient for this nursing practice
- collect and prepare the equipment
- carry out a bowel washout

Related information

Revision of anatomy and physiology of the lower alimentary tract.

Some indications for a bowel washout

A bowel washout is the introduction of fluid through a tube into the rectum and siphoning off the contents to help empty the rectum and sigmoid colon. It is used in the following circumstances:

- prior to special radiological examinations
- prior to sigmoidoscopy
- prior to surgery on the rectum or descending colon
- in certain cases of faecal impaction

Equipment

Trolley or tray
Protective covering for the bed and floor
Disposable gloves
Funnel and tubing or disposable bowel irrigation set (see Fig. 5.9)
Sterile rectal tube – usually Jacques catheter no. 21
Lubricant – KY jelly
Solution as ordered – usually plain water or sodium chloride 0.9%
Medical wipes
Bucket to receive return flow
Receptacle for soiled disposables

Figure 5.9
Disposable bowel irrigation set

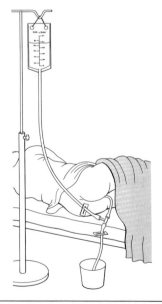

Guidelines for this nursing practice

- explain the nursing practice to the patient and gain his consent and cooperation
- collect and prepare the equipment
- assist the patient into the left lateral position in bed, with his buttocks exposed but ensuring he is adequately covered and has as much privacy as possible
- observe the patient throughout this activity
- place the protective covering on the bed, under the patient's buttocks, and the other protective covering on the floor at the side of the bed, under the bucket which receives the return flow
- join the Jacques catheter to the funnel and tubing
- don the disposable gloves
- lubricate the end of the catheter
- run some of the solution through the tubing and catheter to expel the air

- clamp the end of the catheter before all the solution has run out and then introduce the catheter into the rectum in an upwards and backwards direction for 10–12 cm
- administer 120–150 ml fluid then invert the funnel over the bucket until all the fluid runs back out or close inlet gateclip and open outlet gateclip to allow fluid to run into bucket (see Fig. 5.9)
- observe the character of the return flow
- repeat the practice until the return flow is clear or until all the solution ordered has been used
- gently withdraw the catheter
- dry the perineal area
- remove the protective covering
- ensure the patient is left feeling as comfortable as possible
- dispose of the equipment safely
- document this nursing practice, monitor after-effects and report abnormal findings immediately

Bowel Washout

Maintaining a safe environment

Although this does not require aseptic technique, all the equipment should be clean or disposable. The nurse should wash her hands before commencing and on completion of the practice.

This nursing practice is not usually advised when the patient has rectal bleeding, as the rectal tube may seriously damage an already friable mucosa.

Communicating

A careful explanation of the necessity for this nursing practice should be given to the patient, as he may find it a very embarrassing thing to have done to him.

Eating and drinking

This procedure is often carried out prior to surgery on the bowel. After the procedure the patient may be limited to fluids or to a low residue diet.

Eliminating

Ensure access for the patient to a bedpan, commode or toilet after this nursing practice.

Mobilising

The effectiveness of the washout may be increased if the patient can move around in bed to distribute the solution.

Expressing sexuality

This is a very embarrassing practice for the patient, so an adequate explanation should be given and as much privacy as possible should be provided. Ideally it should be carried out in a treatment room away from other patients and convenient for a toilet.

Suggested reading   Ratcliffe P 1988 Whole gut irrig ˘.on: an acceptable risk? Nursing Times 84(18) May 4: 33–34
Roper N, Logan W, Tierney A 1990 The elements of nursing, 3rd edn. Churchill Livingstone, Edinburgh, pp 198–199

Flatus Tube

Objectives

By the end of this section you should know how to:

- prepare the patient for this nursing practice
- collect and prepare the equipment
- insert a flatus tube

Related information

Revision of the anatomy and physiology of the large intestine.

Some indications for inserting a flatus tube

Flatus is a collection of bowel gas which can gather in the colon and rectum. A flatus tube can be passed per rectum:

- to help relieve abdominal discomfort and distension caused by flatus

This is not a common nursing practice nowadays, although it may still be carried out in gynaecological wards and after abdominal surgery which has involved handling the intestines. It can give considerable relief to some patients.

Equipment

Trolley or tray
Protective covering
Disposable flatus tube (Fig. 5.10)
Bowl of warm water
Water-soluble lubricant
Medical wipes
Tubing attached by a connection to the flatus tube may be required to reach the bowl of water
Disposable gloves
Receptacle for soiled disposables

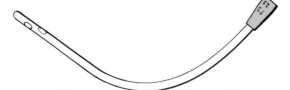

Figure 5.10
Example of a flatus tube

Guidelines for this nursing practice

- explain this nursing practice to the patient and gain his consent and cooperation
- assist the patient into the left lateral position with the buttocks near the edge of the bed
- observe the patient throughout this activity
- place the protective covering under the patient's buttocks
- ensure the patient's privacy
- lubricate the end of the flatus tube and connect it to the tubing if necessary
- put on the disposable gloves

- ensure the end of the tube is under the level of the water in the bowl, which should be at a lower level than the bed
- insert the lubricated end of the tube into the rectum for about 7.5 cm in an upwards and backwards direction following the natural curve of the rectum
- observe the end of the flatus tube which is under water to see if bubbles of gas escape
- remove the tube from the rectum when no more bubbles appear

- dry the anal area
- remove the protective covering
- ensure that the patient is left feeling as comfortable as possible
- dispose of the equipment safely
- document this nursing practice appropriately, monitor after-effects and report abnormal findings immediately

Relevance to the activities of living

Maintaining a safe environment

Although this does not require aseptic technique, the equipment should be clean or disposable. The nurse should wash her hands before commencing and on completion of the nursing practice.

This practice should not be attempted if surgery has involved the rectum or anal area, because of the damage that might be caused to the mucosa by the insertion of the flatus tube.

Communicating

A clear explanation of this nursing practice must be given to the patient, to gain his full cooperation.

Eating and drinking

Educating the patient in the correct sort of diet to choose in the postoperative period can help lessen the discomfort from flatus. The diet should have a high protein and fibre content, but gas-forming foods such as onions, nuts and peas should be avoided.

Mobilising

The patient should be encouraged to move around as much as possible as this helps to disperse the flatus.

Expressing sexuality

This may be an embarrassing practice for the patient, so a clear explanation must be given and as much privacy as possible should be provided.

Suggested reading

Clarke M 1983 Practical nursing. Baillière Tindall, London, pp 162–165, 169
Hamilton H (ed) 1985 Nurse's reference library – procedures. Springhouse Corporation, Pennsylvania, p 581

Stoma Care

Objectives

By the end of this section you should know how to:

- prepare the patient for this nursing practice
- collect and prepare the equipment
- carry out stoma care for the patient
- help the patient accept and care for the stoma himself

Related information

Revision of the anatomy and physiology of the digestive system, with special reference to the small and large intestine.

Review of health board policy regarding the role of the stoma care nurse and the available literature for patient education.

Knowledge of the information and level of counselling given to the patient before the operation to create a stoma.

Some indications for stoma care

A stoma is an opening from the small or large intestine on to the surface of the abdomen through which the bowel contents are diverted for excretion. A stoma is formed following surgical intervention for treatment of intestinal disease. Different names are used according to the site of the stoma.

Stoma care involves cleansing of the stoma and surrounding skin, and the provision of a suitable appliance for the safe collection and disposal of excreta, in order to enable the person to resume normal activities of living as soon as possible.

A *colostomy* is an opening from the colon, usually the transverse or descending colon, and may be required:

- for patients who have malignant disease of the rectum or colon
- for patients who have diverticular disease of the colon
- for patients who have inflammatory disease of the intestine, e.g. Crohn's disease or ulcerative colitis

An *ileostomy* is an opening from the ileum and may be formed for the same reasons as a colostomy, but is more often formed for patients who have inflammatory disease of the intestine, e.g. Crohn's disease or ulcerative colitis.

In some cases a temporary stoma may be formed so that once the disease has resolved, the stoma may be closed and the intestine anastomosed to function as before.

A *jejunostomy* is an opening from the jejunum.

An *urostomy* is an opening from the bladder or ureters into a segment of the ileum which is used as a channel for the urine to be diverted through an abdominal stoma. This is also known as an ileal conduit and may be required for treatment of malignant disease of the bladder.

Equipment

Trolley or tray

A bowl of warm water

Tissues or paper towels

Material for protecting the skin area round the stoma, e.g. Stomahesive, karaya gum

Suitable appliance (stoma bag)

Scissors

Measuring jug

Gloves (non-sterile)

Barrier cream for protecting the skin around the stoma

Deodorant as required

Receptacle for soiled disposables

Stoma appliances

There is a wide range of appliances available and, with the guidance of a stoma care nurse, the patient chooses the one most suitable for his needs. Bags may have pre-cut apertures or they may have to be cut to fit individually. They may be closed pouches or open-ended to allow emptying (Fig. 5.11). Some are two-piece appliances with a semi-rigid circular aperture on which a bag can be clipped, allowing for changing or emptying.

Figure 5.11
Examples of disposable stoma bags
A Closed pouch
B Open lower end to permit emptying of contents

A

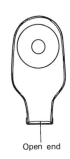

B

Open end

Immediately postoperatively the surgeon will have placed a clear plastic appliance over the stoma, probably incorporating a suitable backing to protect the skin. This allows observation of the stoma and its function. Protective backing also allows removal of the appliance without too much discomfort to the patient during the postoperative period. It may be 2–5 days before the appliance needs to be changed for the first time.

Karaya gum-backed appliance: This appliance may have a circle of karaya gum pre-cut, when the appropriate size to fit the stoma should be chosen; otherwise a hole should be prepared by cutting the karaya backing to a suitable size. The gum must be moistened before applying to the skin (see manufacturer's instructions).

Skin protective wafer, e.g. Stomahesive: This is a square wafer in which a hole is cut to fit snugly round the stoma. A bag with an adhesive backing is prepared to fit over the stoma and adhere to the wafer (see manufacturer's instructions).

Protective cream: Occasionally protective barrier creams or gels may be prescribed for patients who have particularly sensitive skin. These should be massaged into the skin until dry and non-greasy, and any surplus cream wiped off before the new appliance is fitted.

Deodorants: These can range from sprays to concentrated deodorants where only one drop is needed. The stoma care nurse should be consulted about preparations most suitable for the patient's needs.

Guidelines for this nursing practice

- explain the nursing practice to the patient and gain his consent and cooperation
- ensure the patient's privacy
- collect and prepare the equipment
- help the patient into a comfortable position
- help to adjust clothing to expose the patient's abdomen in the area of the stoma
- don gloves
- place a paper towel appropriately to protect the surrounding area from any spills or leakage
- observe the patient throughout this activity
- empty appliance and measure contents if required
- gently remove the appliance and protective backing
- wash the skin around the stoma with warm water only. Soap may cause skin irritation

- encourage the patient to look at his stoma and explain what you are doing
- observe the colour and condition of the stoma and the surrounding skin
- dry the skin around the stoma thoroughly
- prepare the appliance as required by cutting the aperture of the bag and the skin protective wafer if necessary
- apply any prescribed protective creams if required and remove any surplus cream
- place the new appliance in position so that it fits comfortably, and allows no leakage round the stoma (Fig. 5.12)
- seal an open-ended bag with appropriate closure
- ensure that the patient is left feeling as comfortable as possible
- document the nursing practice appropriately, monitor after-effects, and report abnormal findings immediately

Figure 5.12
Positioning an appliance over a stoma
A Removing protective covering from adhesive ring before placing appliance over stoma
B Applying a stoma bag. The open-ended pouch is sealed with a clip ready for use; when the clip is removed, the stoma bag can be emptied without removing the appliance from the skin

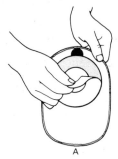

A

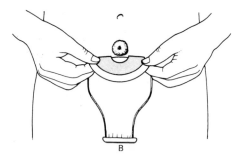

B

Relevance to the activities of living

Maintaining a safe environment

In the postoperative period, the abdominal wound should be dressed separately using aseptic technique, and covered with plastic sealant spray or a sterile dressing, before stoma care is performed (see Aseptic technique, p. 26).

Care of the stoma itself is not a sterile practice, but high standards of cleanliness should be maintained. Stoma care should be regarded as a form of toileting and appropriate hand washing performed. Patient education should reflect this as he is helped to look after his own stoma under the guidance of the stoma care nurse and others involved with his care.

The contents of the stoma bag should be emptied into the toilet or Clinamatic. The soiled bags should be treated as clinical waste. Once home, the patient will be instructed to wrap the bags in newspaper when they have been emptied and rinsed. They should be placed in the dustbin for disposal, although in some health authority areas a special service is available for removal and disposal of soiled bags.

Communicating

An important part of the patient's postoperative care should be to help him care for the stoma himself. It is helpful for all nursing staff to know the level of counselling given to each patient before the operation, and the involvement of the stoma care nurse in this instruction. The nurse should encourage the patient to talk about the stoma, and create an environment for him to ask questions about any worries he has, while performing stoma care for him initially and then while helping him learn to care for the stoma himself. There should be a good liaison between the ward staff and the stoma care nurse, so that the patient feels he can discuss his concerns freely. Literature about his particular type of stoma should be readily available from the stoma care nurse, and discussions can be a useful aid for communication and patient education.

Details of local support groups and a visit from someone successfully coping with a stoma can help the patient with his own adjustment to the stoma.

Initially, the patient may find the smell of flatus and excreta from the stoma difficult to accept. It should be explained that once a normal diet is established he will soon find out which foods appear to make the flatus worse, and exclude them. Once the stoma is established and functioning normally unpleasant odour will be less of a problem. Local deodorant can be used, and some appliances are fitted with deodorant filters to cope with the problem. Advice from the stoma care nurse should be sought. The most important way of helping the patient is for the nurse to indicate by her non-verbal communication that she is not upset by normal bodily function taking place in a different area of the body.

If the patient normally uses spectacles, he should be encouraged to wear them initially to watch while stoma care is performed, and later so that he can see properly to do it himself.

Eating and drinking

Once the patient is allowed a normal diet the stoma will discharge faecal material more frequently. By a process of observation the patient should be encouraged to notice the effect which different foods have on faecal elimination. In this way he may be able to adjust his diet so that a more solid stool is formed. This process may take several weeks and the stoma care nurse will continue to give help and advice about appropriate diet when the patient is at home.

Relevance to the
activities of living
continued

Eliminating

The presence of a stoma completely changes the way in which faecal material is eliminated from the body and the patient has to be helped to adjust to this.

Preoperatively the patient should be involved with the discussion and decision of the site for his stoma. The stoma care nurse, the surgeon and the ward nursing staff should all be involved with this important preoperative preparation, in their appropriate roles.

In the immediate postoperative period, the patient has no control over faecal material eliminated through a stoma and this is an added problem about which he has to learn. Initially faecal material is fluid when expelled through the stoma, as the water absorption function of the colon may have been bypassed. After 2–3 weeks, when the patient is able to eat a normal diet, a semisolid stool may be formed, especially when the stoma is a colostomy in the transverse or descending colon. Eventually the frequency of bowel function can be reduced and controlled and almost resemble normal bowel movement, to the extent that a stoma bag need not be worn continuously.

Drainage from an ileostomy, on the other hand, is liquid and rich in digestive enzymes which can cause excoriation and erosion of the skin. The discharge flows almost continuously, requiring constant wear of an appliance unless an ileal pouch (a reservoir below the skin surface) has been constructed. Odour problems, fear of soiling and skin complications are more common with an ileostomy, and an open-ended bag which can be emptied regularly is the most suitable appliance. Eventually, however, there is usually some control over the frequency of bowel function.

Appliances should be emptied or changed as often as necessary to prevent over-filling and leakage on to the surrounding skin area (usually $\frac{1}{3} - \frac{1}{2}$ full or they become heavy and unwieldy). Any redness, swelling or abnormalities of the stoma or the surrounding skin area should be reported.

Initially, the faecal fluid should be measured and observed for any abnormalities. Abnormal excreta should be kept for observation and reported.

An urostomy is formed to allow urine to be excreted through an abdominal stoma. This may be collected directly into a suitable stoma bag, or a catheter may be incorporated so that a closed drainage system may be used. Whichever system is used the bag chosen should have facilities for frequent emptying (see catheter care p. 212). The principles of stoma care remain the same.

Personal cleansing and dressing

The patient may feel that the stoma is a threat to his cleanliness. Shower or bathing facilities should be available as soon as his condition allows and prior to that a bed bath given as often as required. Stoma care should be coordinated with showering or bathing whenever possible; the appliance can be emptied and removed and the skin area washed first, and the new appliance fitted afterwards. This may not be possible with an ileostomy or urostomy, and in these instances the appliance should be emptied, or changed and replaced, before showering or bathing.

While the patient is learning how to care for the stoma, comfortable clothes which give easy access to the stoma should be worn. Modern appliances are comfortable and unobtrusive so no permanent change in clothing style should be needed. Advice from the stoma care nurse and the appropriate support group can be helpful.

Working and playing

Once the patient has recovered from the operation and is able to cope with the stoma it is hoped that he will return to his normal lifestyle. Even swimming is possible, using a small temporary appliance. Helpful advice can be obtained from the stoma care nurse and support groups.

Expressing sexuality

A stoma, especially if it is permanent, is a major insult to the patient's body image and he may become withdrawn and depressed. His acceptance by the hospital staff will be the first step in giving the patient confidence in himself. He should choose which of his friends and relatives he tells about the stoma, and their acceptance will help his rehabilitation. Counselling before the operation and constant support from all concerned will boost his morale, and help him overcome the almost inevitable initial revulsion.

Patients who have stoma following resection of the lower bowel may have problems with sexual function. Men may become impotent, and women may have dyspareunia, and sexual partners should be included in counselling before and after surgery. Inevitably the presence of an abdominal stoma appliance calls for additional thoughtfulness and ingenuity during sexual intercourse. Counselling from the stoma care nurse, the surgeon and the appropriate support group will help in this situation, which may only be temporary.

Sleeping

Stoma care should be performed prior to the patient settling for the night, as this will prevent the need to empty or change an appliance and thus disturb sleep. Once the patient is eating a normal diet, and has adjusted to his own requirements, it is unlikely that the stoma will need any attention during the night. A larger bag can be used overnight, which may be helpful for patients who have an ileostomy.

Suggested reading

Ball J 1989 Educating for stoma care. Nursing Times 85(34) August 23: 54–55
Bell N 1989 Sexuality and the ostomist. Nursing Times 85(5) February 1: 28–30
Bradley C 1990 The role of the stoma care nurse. Nursing 4(18) September 13: 9–11
Davis K 1990 Impotence after surgery. Nursing 4(18) September 13: 23–25
Donaldson I 1989 Communication can help the ostomist to accept their stoma. Professional Nurse 4(5) February: 242–244
Elcoat C 1988 Stoma care. Taking a holistic approach. Nursing Times 84(9) March: 57–60
Foulkes B Understanding colostomy (A handbook for patients). Squibb Surgicare Limited, Hounslow, Middlesex
Horsfield Gardiner J 1987 Asians in Britain. Some cultural considerations in stoma care. Nursing 3(21) September: 785–789
Model G 1990 A new image to accept. Psychological aspects of stoma care. Professional Nurse 5(6) March: 310–316
Reed A 1989 Attitudes to stoma patients. Nursing Times 85(17) April 26: 65, 67–70, 72
Roper N, Logan W, Tierney A 1990 The elements of nursing, 3rd edn. Churchill Livingstone, Edinburgh, pp 194–201
Wade B 1990 A stoma is for life. Scutari Press, London

Abdominal Paracentesis

Objectives

By the end of this section you should know how to:

- prepare the patient for this procedure
- collect and prepare the equipment
- assist the medical practitioner with abdominal paracentesis as required

Related information

Revision of the anatomy and physiology of the abdominal organs, with special reference to the peritoneum.

Revision of aseptic technique (see p. 26).

Some indications for abdominal paracentesis

Abdominal paracentesis is the removal of fluid from the peritoneal cavity through a sterile cannula or needle. Sometimes medication may be introduced into the peritoneal cavity by the same route.

This procedure may be performed for the following reasons:

- to obtain a specimen of abdominal fluid for diagnostic purposes
- to relieve intra-abdominal pressure caused by increased fluid within the abdominal cavity. This symptom is called ascites and may occur in association with several conditions, e.g.:
  — patients who have congestive cardiac failure involving dysfunction of the right side of the heart
  — patients who have chronic hepatic disease
  — patients who have malignant disease with metastases in the liver
- to introduce medication into the peritoneal cavity, e.g.
  — cytotoxic therapy for malignant disease

Outline of the procedure

Abdominal paracentesis is carried out by the medical practitioner using aseptic technique. A mask and sterile gown as well as sterile gloves should be worn.

The site of insertion is midway between the umbilicus and the symphysis pubis along the midline.

The skin is cleaned with antiseptic lotion and a local anaesthetic is administered. The area round the site is covered with sterile towels. A small skin incision is made with a sterile blade and a trocar and cannula are inserted into the peritoneal cavity. The trocar is removed, allowing fluid to flow through the cannula. Required specimens of abdominal fluid for investigation are collected at this stage by holding the appropriately labelled sterile containers under the flow of fluid, maintaining asepsis. The cannula may be removed and a sterile dressing applied, or it may be stitched in position and attached to sterile tubing and a closed drainage bag, if drainage is to be maintained. A suitable sterile dressing should be applied round the cannula. The flow of drainage fluid is regulated with a gate clamp or roller clamp to prevent too rapid a reduction of intra-abdominal pressure. Initially only 1 l of fluid should be allowed to drain before regulating the flow to 100 ml per hour, or as prescribed by the medical practitioner.

Equipment

Trolley
Theatre mask
Sterile gown
Sterile gloves
Sterile dressings pack
Sterile towels
Sterile bowl
Sterile specimen containers appropriately labelled, completed laboratory forms and a plastic specimen bag for transportation
Antiseptic lotion
Sterile abdominal paracentesis set containing:
— specialised trocar and cannula
— forceps
— blade and holder
— tubing
Local anaesthetic and equipment for its administration
Sterile sutures and needle for stitching the cannula in position
Sterile drainage bag
Gate clip or roller clamp
Disposable tape measure
Measuring jug
Receptacle for soiled disposables

Abdominal Paracentesis

Guidelines for this nursing practice

- help to explain the procedure to the patient and gain his consent and cooperation
- ask the patient to empty his bladder immediately prior to the procedure. This will ensure that the bladder remains within the pelvis, so preventing any risk of perforation when the trocar is inserted
- ensure the patient's privacy
- measure and record the patient's abdominal girth before commencing the procedure
- help collect and prepare the equipment
- help the patient into a suitable, comfortable position. He may sit upright with his back well supported. If possible the legs may be lowered to allow easier access to the insertion site and to increase the patient's comfort. A bed which can be adjusted to allow just the lower limbs to be lowered is the most suitable. In some instances the medical practitioner may prefer that the patient lies flat. The chosen position depends on the reason for the abdominal paracentesis

- help to adjust the patient's clothing to expose the site of insertion
- observe the patient throughout this activity
- help to prepare the sterile field as required
- assist the medical practitioner as required during the procedure
- measure the amount of drainage and adjust the flow of drainage fluid as required
- ensure that the patient is left feeling as comfortable as possible in a sitting position, so that drainage is encouraged
- dispose of equipment safely
- dispatch labelled specimens of abdominal fluid to the appropriate laboratory with their completed forms immediately
- document the procedure appropriately, monitor after-effects and report abnormal findings immediately

Relevance to the activities of living

Maintaining a safe environment

This is an invasive procedure giving direct access to the peritoneal cavity so all precautions to minimise the risk of infection should be maintained. Asepsis should be maintained and adequate hand washing technique should be practised.

Following the procedure, the site should be observed for any redness or swelling which may indicate infection, and this should be reported immediately.

Dressings should be changed as required, using aseptic technique (see Wound care p. 26).

Any leakage of fluid round the cannula should be noted and reported as this may indicate that the cannula is blocked or dislodged.

Safety of staff transporting specimens should be maintained by enclosing containers in plastic specimen bags (see Specimen collection, p. 198).

Communicating

Patients do not normally find this procedure too uncomfortable, even during a period of continuous drainage. When the abdominal paracentesis is performed to relieve pressure caused by excess fluid in the peritoneal cavity, the patient is much more comfortable after the procedure is performed. A prescribed analgesic medication should be administered if required.

Breathing

The patient's blood pressure, pulse and respirations should be recorded 4-hourly following this procedure for 24–48 hours. The frequency of the recordings will depend on the patient's condition and the reason for the abdominal paracentesis.

The blood pressure and pulse should be recorded every half hour for 2 hours immediately following this procedure, when a patient has had severe ascites with a raised intra-abdominal pressure. A sudden drop in this pressure could cause cardiogenic shock due to rapid vasodilation. A low blood pressure recording should be reported immediately and the rate of flow of the drainage fluid should be reduced to a minimum. Initially only 1 l of fluid should be removed before regulating the flow as prescribed by the medical practitioner. This may be 50–150 ml an hour, depending on the patient's condition.

Eating and drinking

Fluid intake should be recorded and accurate fluid balance charts maintained. This will enable any reduction or increase in peritoneal fluid to be monitored in relation to the fluid intake and urinary output.

The appetite may have been poor due to the feeling of fullness and discomfort caused by the ascites; patients often experience indigestion due to pressure on the stomach. Depending on the situation, they may have to be encouraged to eat following this procedure, as protein is lost with the peritoneal fluid. Advice from the dietician may help with the choice of nourishing foods and the family may be encouraged to help provide favourite treats if appropriate.

Abdominal Paracentesis

Relevance to the
activities of living
continued

Eliminating

The colour and viscosity of the peritoneal fluid should be noted. The presence of blood should be noted and reported, as it may indicate some trauma to the abdominal organs during the insertion of the trocar.

The amount of fluid drained should be accurately measured and recorded, and fluid balance charts should be maintained throughout this procedure. Appropriate arrangements for measuring the urine should be made with the patient's cooperation. The patient may be helped to the toilet, or to use a commode, depending on his condition.

Fluids and electrolytes pass across the peritoneal membrane, so electrolytes may also be lost in the drained ascitic fluid. This could cause hypokalaemia (low potassium levels) or hyponatraemia (low sodium levels). The medical practitioner will monitor the patient's blood chemistry and prescribe replacement potassium and sodium as required. The loss of protein may also be a concern, as this is often present in ascitic fluid.

Drainage of large amounts of excess peritoneal fluid is not performed routinely, as the fluid will reform from the circulation unless the cause itself can be treated. Amounts sufficient to relieve distressing pressure and associated symptoms can be removed without causing problems.

When ascites is caused by abdominal metastases the patient may gain some relief from continuous drainage of the excess peritoneal fluid, and this will be prescribed as appropriate.

The measurement of the abdominal girth may help to monitor developing or improving ascites. The bladder should be emptied before the daily measurement which should be taken at the same position each time. To facilitate accurate measurement, and with the patient's permission, lines may be drawn on each side of the abdomen outlining the path of the tape measure for 1 or 2 cm.

Peritoneal dialysis: A form of abdominal paracentesis is used as one of the treatments for renal failure. Continuous ambulatory peritoneal dialysis (CAPD) uses the properties of the peritoneal membrane as a substitute kidney. A permanent catheter is inserted into the peritoneal cavity. A quantity of sterile dialysis fluid is introduced through the catheter where it remains in the peritoneal cavity for 4 hours. The fluid is then allowed to drain out over half an hour. This procedure is repeated continuously over 24 hours, so that nitrogenous waste and excess electrolytes can be eliminated from the body.

The patient may be taught how to introduce his own dialysis fluid and drain the peritoneal fluid using aseptic technique. This method of home dialysis allows the patient to continue a relatively normal lifestyle.

Personal cleansing and dressing

Depending on the patient's condition he may be able to have a shower while this procedure is in progress, and a waterproof dressing can be used to protect the cannula site.

The patient's clothes may have to be adapted to accommodate the cannula and drainage bag.

Controlling body temperature

The temperature should be recorded 4-hourly during and following this procedure to monitor any change in body temperature which might indicate a developing infection. Any abnormality should be reported immediately.

Mobilising

Immediately following this procedure the patient should remain in bed to enable observations of his condition to be maintained. Mobilising may then be encouraged as his condition allows. Patients with a continuous drainage system may need help to maintain a safe environment when mobilising, to prevent infection or disconnection of the tubing. Patients treated with continuous ambulatory peritoneal dialysis (CAPD) for chronic renal failure may roll up their empty bag and tuck it under their waist band once the dialysis fluid is in situ, and then recommence normal activities.

Expressing sexuality

The presence of an abdominal catheter will present the patient with a feeling of an altered body image. The nurse's attitude and communication skills, both verbal and non-verbal, can help the patient to accept this. The relief of abdominal pressure from excess ascites should help the patient's acceptance. Patients on CAPD should be counselled with their sexual partners. They should be encouraged to seek guidance from local support groups.

Suggested reading Roper N, Logan W, Tierney A 1990 The elements of nursing, 3rd edn. Churchill Livingstone, Edinburgh, pp 194–201
Ryan E, Neale G 1981 Procedure in practice. Devonshire Press, Torquay, pp 7–9
Stanfield G 1985 Coping with CAPD. Nursing Mirror 16(14) October 2: 28–29
Strangio L 1988 Believe it or not, peritoneal dialysis made easy. Nursing (US) 18(1) January: 43–46
Young M E et al 1988 Third spacing. When a body conceals fluid loss. RN 51(8) August: 46–48

Personal Cleansing and Dressing

Bathing and Showering

Objectives

By the end of this section you should know how to:

- prepare the patient for this nursing practice
- collect and prepare the equipment
- help the patient with an immersion bath or shower

Related information

Revision of the anatomy and physiology of the skin with special reference to its function as a barrier to infection.

Review of local policy regarding preoperative skin preparation.

Review of health authority policy regarding cleaning bathroom equipment and control of infection.

Some indications for immersion bath or shower

An immersion bath or shower enables the patient to have a total body wash, and may be indicated:

- to maintain personal hygiene and promote a feeling of well-being
- to clean the skin prior to surgery in order to help prevent infection in the wound area during the operation
- to clean the skin following surgery to prevent infection and promote healing

Equipment

Soap
Face cloth
Bath towel
Clean clothing
Chosen toiletries, e.g. talcum powder, perfume, aftershave
Suitable bath or shower
A chair or shower stool
Disposable floor mat

Guidelines for this nursing practice

Bathing

- discuss the arrangements for his bath with the patient and gain his consent and cooperation
- help the patient collect and prepare the equipment
- help the patient to the bathroom; this may include the use of mechanical lifting aids or a wheelchair
- ensure the patient's privacy
- prepare the water in the bath maintaining a safe temperature and gain the patient's approval
- help the patient to undress
- observe the patient throughout this activity
- help the patient into the bath. For some patients, two nurses may be needed to help the patient, or mechanical aids may be used according to the manufacturer's instructions
- help the patient to wash himself, commencing with washing and drying his face and neck (see Bed bath p. 250)
- help to wash the patient's hair if required (see Hair care p. 262)

- help the patient out of the bath. He may sit on a chair which is protected with a towel to prevent any unsteadiness
- help the patient to dry himself as required
- help to apply talcum powder if required
- help the patient to dress himself
- allow the patient time to clean his teeth or dentures at the basin, giving help as required
- help to brush or comb the patient's hair
- help the patient to a chair or bed as he chooses, or as his condition allows
- ensure that the patient is left feeling as comfortable as possible
- clean the bath
- dispose of equipment safely
- document the nursing practice appropriately, monitor after-effects and report abnormal findings immediately

Showering

- discuss the arrangements for his shower with the patient and gain his consent and cooperation
- help collect and prepare the equipment
- help the patient to the shower room. This may include the use of mechanical lifting aids or a wheelchair
- help the patient to undress
- help the patient to sit on the shower chair or stool

- adjust the flow of water from the shower to maintain a safe water temperature and gain the patient's approval
- help the patient to wash himself while showering
- help the patient to wash his hair if required
- help the patient to dry himself
- proceed as for Guidelines for bathing

Bathing and Showering

Relevance to the activities of living

Maintaining a safe environment

The nurse should ensure that the patient has appropriate assistance to help him bath or shower safely.

A chair should be available so that he can sit to dry or dress himself to prevent any danger of falling.

The water temperature should be checked to ensure that there is no danger of scalding. The ability to judge temperature may be impaired in elderly patients, or those with diabetic neuropathy, so the water temperature should always be checked by a nurse or a responsible adult. The use of a bath thermometer will help with this.

The bath or shower area should be cleaned after each use. If the nurse is not confident that this has been done the bath should be cleaned before preparing it for the patient, to prevent any cross-infection.

Communicating

As far as possible the choice and timing of a bath or shower should be arranged according to the patient's preference. However the patient's condition and the ward situation may affect this, and appropriate arrangements should be discussed with the patient to gain his cooperation.

The development of a caring relationship between the nurse and the patient is often enhanced when bathing or showering a patient. The opportunity for communication is increased and the nurse can encourage the patient to talk about himself, his family or his worries, and this information may contribute to the nursing assessment. The time can also be used for patient education in relation to personal hygiene, using good communication skills.

Eliminating

The patient should be given the opportunity to use the toilet or commode before bathing or showering.

Personal cleansing and dressing

While bathing the patient the nurse should observe the condition of his skin for any abnormalities. Any redness, rashes, bruises, sores or lumps should be noted and reported (see Bed bath, p. 250).

The skin should be dried carefully after bathing or showering, especially in the creases of the body, e.g. under the breasts and in the groin. This helps to maintain the skin in good condition as a barrier to infection. A light dusting with talcum powder may help to keep the skin dry, but too much may collect in the body creases and cause soreness.

If possible the patient should be encouraged to wear his own clothes after a bath or shower to help retain his individuality.

Controlling body temperature

The bath or shower room should be at a comfortable room temperature of 18–21°C. This will prevent loss of body heat after a bath, when the patient may be exposed during drying and dressing.

Mobilising

Mechanical lifting aids should be used appropriately, according to the manufacturer's instructions, to help the patient in and out of a bath or shower.

Expressing sexuality

If the patient is left alone to bath and shower, it is often difficult to ensure the safety of his environment and complete privacy, but patients usually accept the help of the nurse if the reason is explained. The nurse's attitude and communication skills should help acceptance of this invasion of privacy and prevent embarrassment. Apart from necessary attendant helpers, privacy should be ensured during this activity.

Male patients should be encouraged or helped to shave before or immediately after bathing or showering. They may like to apply some pleasant after shave lotion to enhance their self image.

Women may be encouraged to apply make-up and perfume after bathing to help their individuality and self-esteem.

Suggested reading

Gilchrist B 1990 Washing and dressing after surgery. Nursing Times 86(50) December 12: 71

Gooch J 1987 Skin hygiene. Professional Nurse 2(5) February: 153–154

Kalideen D 1990 Preparing skin for surgery. Nursing 4(15) July 26: 28–29

Roper N, Logan W, Tierney A 1990 The elements of nursing, 3rd edn. Churchill Livingstone, Edinburgh, pp 202–229

Tierney A (ed) 1986 Clinical nursing practice. Recent advances in nursing 14. Churchill Livingstone, Edinburgh, pp 154–184

Walsh M, Ford P 1989 Nursing rituals; research and rational actions. Heinemann Nursing, Oxford pp 16–18, 114

Webster R et al 1988 Patients' and nurses' opinions about bathing. Nursing Times (occasional paper) 84(37) September 14: 54–57

Bed Bath

Objectives

By the end of this section you should know how to:

- prepare the patient for this nursing practice
- collect the equipment
- carry out a bed bath

Related information

Revision of the anatomy and physiology of the skin tissue, skin care.

Revision of skin care (see p. 256) and mouth care (see p. 268).

Some indications for a bed bath

Bed bathing is assisting a bedfast patient to maintain his personal hygiene during his period of bedrest. A patient may require a bed bath:

- postoperatively following major surgery when mobility is restricted
- following an acute illness, e.g. myocardial infarction
- while in an unconscious state
- following trauma, e.g. a patient in traction
- when a patient is extremely weak and debilitated due to the prolonged effects of a disease, trauma or treatment being administered

Equipment

Basin of hot water (35–40°C)
Lotion thermometer
Soap, preferably the patient's own
Patient's toiletries such as deodorant, talcum powder
Bath towels, preferably the patient's own
Two face cloths or sponges
Disposable paper towel or similar
Patient's brush and comb
Nail scissors and nail file if required
Clean nightdress or pyjamas
Clean bed linen
Trolley
Equipment for catheter care (see p. 212) if required
Equipment for skin care (see p. 256)
Equipment for mouth care (see p. 268)
Receptacle for soiled patient clothing
Receptacle for soiled bed linen
Receptacle for soiled disposables

Guidelines for this nursing practice

- explain the nursing practice to the patient and gain his consent and cooperation
- collect and prepare the equipment
- ensure the patient's privacy
- observe the patient throughout this activity
- check the bed brakes are in use
- help the patient into a comfortable position
- arrange the furniture around the patient's bed space to allow easy access to equipment on the trolley
- remove excess bed linen and bed appliances if in use, but leaving the patient covered with a bed sheet
- help the patient remove his pyjamas or gown
- check the temperature of the basin of water using the lotion thermometer
- ask the patient to test the water temperature

- check with the patient if he uses soap on his face
- wash, rinse and dry the patient's face, ears and neck; when possible assist the patient to do this for himself
- expose only the part of the patient's body being washed
- change the water as it cools, becomes dirty or immediately after washing the patient's pubic area
- wash, rinse and dry thoroughly the patient's body in an appropriate order such as the upper limbs, chest and abdomen, back, lower limbs, and anal area
- when washing the patient's limbs, wash first the limb furthest away from you. This will allow the assistant to dry that limb as the other limb is washed, thus reducing the time the patient's body is exposed to the cooling effect of the environment. When possible assist the patient to immerse his feet and hands in the basin of water (Fig. 6.1)

Figure 6.1
Foot immersion: the patient's foot and leg should be supported. Upper limbs can be supported in a similar way

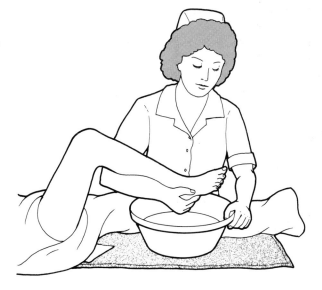

Guidelines for this
nursing practice
continued

- as each part of the patient's body is washed, observe the skin for any blemish, redness or discoloration which can alert the nurse to the potential problem of pressure sore development (see Skin care p 256)

- apply body deodorants and/or talcum powder as desired by the patient

- assist the patient to wash, rinse and dry his pubic area using the extra face cloth/sponge or the disposable paper towel, washing from the front of the perineal area to the back to prevent cross-infection from the anal region (Fig. 6.2)

- carry out catheter care if required (see p. 212)

- help the patient to dress in his clean pyjamas or gown

- assist the patient to cut and clean his finger- and toenails if required, unless otherwise instructed

- remake the patient's bed

- assist the patient with his mouth care (see p. 268)

- assist the patient to brush or comb his hair into its usual style

- ensure that the patient is left feeling as comfortable as possible

- rearrange the furniture as wished by the patient so that articles he requires are within easy reach

- dispose of the equipment safely

- document the nursing practice appropriately, monitor after-effects and report any abnormal findings immediately

Figure 6.2
Perineal hygiene: wash in one direction only from front to back of perineum

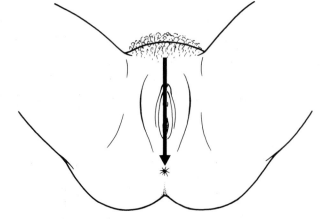

Relevance to the activities of living

Maintaining a safe environment

It is necessary to wash at regular intervals to keep the natural flora of microorganisms within manageable limits. When a patient is confined to bed, a bed bath is one of the nursing practices used to reduce the potential problem of cross-infection or infection of the patient himself during the period of vulnerability due to illness.

The nurse must check that the temperature of the water is at a safe level prior to starting the bed bath and maintain this temperature throughout the bath to assist with patient comfort. The water should be changed as it becomes dirty, cooler or immediately following perineal hygiene. When assisting the patient with perineal hygiene, wash from front to back to reduce the problem of cross-infection from the anal region.

All equipment used should be clean or disposable and all precautions be taken to prevent cross-infection. The nurse should wash her hands before commencing and on completion of a bed bath.

It is preferable that the patient has a personal washbasin during his period of hospitalisation. The nurse should wash the basin and trolley with a detergent and water solution, drying thoroughly prior to and following a bed bath. The basin should be clean and dry when not in use and stored at the patient's bedside, possibly behind the locker.

The patient's face cloth or sponge should be rinsed in clean water, returned to the patient's locker along with the other toilet items used and any soiled personal patient clothing which relatives wish to take home for laundering. Any appliances removed during the bed bath, such as a bed cage, bed table or cot sides, should be returned to their previous position.

Communicating

The nurse and patient should engage in verbal communication during a bed bath but this may require to be kept to a minimum when a patient is acutely ill. When a patient is acutely ill or unconscious, non-verbal cues can be used as a method of communication between the nurse and patient; touch becomes of increased importance.

The nurse should check that the patient who is suffering pain has had recent pain relief prior to starting a bed bath, as the movement during the bath may exacerbate the pain.

Breathing

Patient movement during a bed bath should be kept to a minimum especially when a patient suffers from dyspnoea; for example, changing the bottom sheet should be planned to minimise movement and effort if the patient is acutely ill. When oxygen therapy is being administered, this can be removed for facial cleansing, hair care and mouth care at separate intervals during the bed bath.

Eliminating

The patient should be offered facilities to empty his bladder prior to commencement of a bed bath.

Bed Bath

Relevance to the
activities of living
continued

Personal cleansing and dressing

A patient who does not wash on a regular basis may require some assistance and education by the nurse as to the benefit of this practice while in hospital and following discharge.

Disposable toiletries are available in all ward areas for patients who may have been admitted as an emergency, until their own personal equipment is brought from home.

Soap should be used with caution as it has a drying effect on the skin. A patient who has dry skin may have an emollient prescribed by a medical practitioner which is added to the water for washing. The patient's skin must be rinsed well and thoroughly dried during the bed bath.

When possible the patient should be dressed in his own bed clothing for his comfort and to help maintain his individuality.

A patient who has the power, movement or sensation of a limb altered temporarily or permanently, such as caused by the position of an intravenous infusion or following a cerebral vascular accident, will require some assistance and education on how to dress and undress during a bed bath. The weak or affected limb is dressed first and undressed last.

The nurse should carry out skin care (see p. 256) during a bed bath.

The patient should be assisted to keep his finger- and toenails clean and manicured. A chiropody service may be available for all patients, but should be used when special care has to be taken of a patient's nails, for instance with a diabetic patient or a patient suffering from peripheral vascular disease, to prevent injury to the nail or nailbed. The nurse may assist the patient to apply nail polish if desired.

When a patient is confined to bed the friction between his head and pillow can cause the hair to become tangled and matted. A patient's hair should be brushed and combed into the usual style during a bed bath and at regular intervals throughout the day to prevent the hair becoming tangled and causing the patient discomfort. The patient can have his hair washed while in bed (see p. 262) to maintain its cleanliness. Should a patient be confined to bed over a prolonged period a hairdresser or barber may be required to cut his hair and style it to improve morale.

Mouth care (see p. 268) may be required during a bed bath.

Controlling body temperature

Before commencing the bed bath the nurse should check that the environment around the patient's bed space is at a comfortable temperature and no draughts are evident. During the bed bath the nurse should ensure that the patient is kept warm, as excessive loss of body heat could lead to the patient becoming hypothermic.

Expressing sexuality

Within western society, to feel fresh and clean is known to create a positive body image and maintain self-esteem. Therefore, as well as feeling more comfortable, a patient confined to bed will also benefit psychologically from a bed bath.

When possible assist the patient to maintain individuality and independence by allowing him to wash and dry any part of his body such as his face, hands and pubic area. As the patient has no choice in the method used for cleansing, allow him to make what other choices are available, such as which clothing he wishes to wear. The use of a body deodorant, perfume and make-up are personal traits, and the nurse should be guided by the patient in their application.

Suggested reading

Ayliffe G, Collins B, Taylor L 1982 Hospital acquired infection: principles and prevention. J. Wright, Bristol

Croton C 1990 Duvets on trial. Nursing Times 86(26) June 27: 63–67

Davidson L 1989 Patient clothing: time for a change. Nursing Times 85(48) November 29: 26–29

Gooch J 1987 Skin hygiene. The Professional Nurse 2(5) February: 153–154

Greaves A 1985 We'll just freshen you up dear ... . Nursing Times Journal of Infection Control Nursing 81(10) March 6: 3–8 (Investigation into the misuse of patient wash bowls)

Roper N, Logan W, Tierney A 1990 The elements of nursing, 3rd edn. Churchill Livingstone, Edinburgh, pp 202–218

Turnbull P 1985 Clothes for independence. Nursing Times 81(46) November 13: 55

Webster O, Cowan M, Allen J 1986 Dirty linen. Nursing Times 82(44) October 29: 36–37 (Advantages of using duvets to reduce cross-infection)

Webster R, Thompson D, Bowman G, Sutton T 1988 Patients' and Nurses' opinions about bathing: Nursing Times 84(37) September 14: 54–57

Wright L 1990 Bathing by towel (describes new technique). Nursing Times 86(4) January 24: 36–39

Skin Care

Objectives

By the end of this section you should know how to:

- prepare the patient for this nursing practice
- collect the equipment
- carry out skin care

Related information

Revision of the anatomy and physiology of the skin.

Revision of the predisposing factors for development of a pressure sore.

The health authority policy regarding the mechanical aids available to relieve pressure and pressure sore treatments should be reviewed.

Revision of lifting, turning and moving a patient (p. 292) and active and passive exercises (p. 298).

Some indications for skin care

This care involves the maintenance of a patient's skin continuity by ensuring skin cleanliness, relieving skin capillary pressure, ensuring adequate nutritional status and monitoring of potential problems. Skin care is indicated for every patient, but specific circumstances increase the need for care when:

- a patient is incontinent
- a patient's mobility is impaired temporarily or permanently e.g. bedfast, paralysed or unconscious patient
- a patient has a poor nutritional status
- a patient has impaired peripheral circulation

Equipment

Mechanical aid for pressure relief, if used

Guidelines for this nursing practice

- explain the nursing practice to the patient and gain his consent and cooperation

- ensure the patient's privacy

- observe the patient throughout this activity

- assess the risk factor of the patient developing a pressure sore, utilising one of the assessment scales such as the Norton Scale (Fig. 6.3) or Waterlow Scale (Fig. 6.4) (p. 258). This should be performed on admission and when a patient's condition deteriorates

- identify individual patient problem areas, such as a patient with peripheral vascular disease whose affected limb may be at greater risk than the rest of his body

- when a risk factor is noted, institute preventive skin care

- relieve the pressure exerted on the skin surface by regular changes in the patient's body position. Support the patient's body and limbs in natural positions and maintain joint and muscle movement with passive and active exercises (p. 298). A patient who is assessed as having a high risk factor will require pressure relief of the skin at 2-hourly or more frequent intervals

- reduce the pressure on the skin by the use of any of the numerous mechanical aids available such as a sheepskin, heel and elbow pads, Spenco mattress, Mecanaid Netbed, Clinitron bed

- cleanse the skin of an incontinent patient or a patient who is perspiring profusely as required. Use soap with caution as the alkaline content tends to dry the skin and deplete it of its natural oils

- thoroughly dry the skin by patting gently. These measures will decrease the numbers of skin microorganisms

- examine the patient's skin during the nursing practice for signs of redness or loss of integrity

- reduce shearing and friction forces exerted on a patient's skin by utilising a skilled lifting technique when repositioning him, and proper positioning of the patient to prevent him from sliding down in the bed or chair

- maintain or improve, when appropriate, the patient's nutritional status using the services of a dietician if necessary

- educate the patient about preventive care for pressure sore development when his condition permits, e.g. a patient nursed in traction can assist in pressure relief measures. If a patient is at risk of development of pressure sores following discharge from hospital, the nurse may also require to educate the patient's relatives

- following any of the care above, ensure the patient is left feeling as comfortable as possible

- dispose of equipment safely, if used

- document the nursing practice appropriately, monitor after-effects and report abnormal findings immediately

Skin Care

Figure 6.3
Norton Scale (Reproduced with permission from Roper N, Logan W, Tierney A 1985 The elements of nursing, 2nd edn. Churchill Livingstone, Edinburgh)

		A Physical Condition		B Mental condition		C Activity		D Mobility		E Incontinent		Total Score
		Good	4	Alert	4	Ambulant	4	Full	4	Not	4	
		Fair	3	Apathetic	3	Walk/help	3	Sl. limited	3	Occasionally	3	
		Poor	2	Confused	2	Chairbound	2	V. limited	2	Usually/ur.	2	
Name	Date	V. bad	1	Stuporous	1	Bedfast	1	Immobile	1	Doubly	1	

Instructions for use

1. Identify the most appropriate description of the patient (4, 3, 2, 1) under each of the five headings (A to E) and total the result.

2. Record the 'score' with its date in the patient's notes or on a chart.

3. Assess weekly and whenever any change in the patient's condition and/or circumstances.

With a 'score' of 14 and below the patient is 'At Risk' denoting need for intensive care, i.e. 1–2 hourly changes of posture and the use of pressure-relieving aids.

Note: When oedema of the sacral area has been present a rise of score above 14 does not indicate less risk of a lesion.

Figure 6.4
Waterlow Scale

Build/weight for height		Visual skin type		Continence		Mobility		Sex Age		Appetite	
Average	0	Healthy	0	Complete	0	Fully mobile	0	Male	1	Average	0
Above average	2	Tissue paper	1	Occasionally	1	Restricted/	1	Female	2	Poor	1
Below average	3	Dry	1	incontinent		difficult		14–49	1	Anorectic	2
		Oedematous	1	Catheter/	2	Restless/	2	50–64	2		
		Clammy	1	incontinent		fidgety		65–75	3		
		Discolour	2	of faeces		Apathetic	3	75–80	4		
		Broken/spot	3	Doubly incontinent	3	Inert/traction	4	81+	5		

Special risk factors:

(1) Poor nutrition eg terminal cachexia	8	
(2) Sensory deprivation eg diabetes, paraplegia, cerebrovascular accident	5	**Assessment value**
(3) High dose anti-inflammatory or steroids in use	3	At-risk = 10
(4) Smoking 10+ per day	1	High risk = 15
(5) Orthopaedic surgery/fracture below waist	3	Very high risk = 20

Directions for use:

1 Assess the patient, circling the number in each category in which the patient fits
2 Add up all the numbers, including 'special risk factors'
3 If the total places the patient within the 'at risk', 'high risk' or 'very high risk' areas, turn the card over and read the suggested preventive aids listed on the back
4 Record the circled numbers in the patient's documentation, giving the total and the date
5 Assess each patient every third day, unless the need to reassess the patient earlier becomes evident

Relevance to the activities of living

Maintaining a safe environment

All equipment should be clean or disposable and all precautions be taken to prevent cross-infection. The nurse should wash her hands before commencing, and on completion of, the nursing practice.

Equipment which is used to relieve pressure must be checked at regular intervals to maintain its working condition. The equipment should be kept clean and dry both when in use and when in storage, to reduce microbial growth, which could act as a source of infection to the patient.

If a pressure sore develops, cleansing and dressing of this wound must involve aseptic technique (see p. 26). A sore is a break in skin continuity and is therefore at risk of infection. There are numerous dressing materials and agents available. The dressing of choice should be one which will provide maximum patient comfort and promote wound healing.

Sensory impairment to the skin may predispose to the development of a pressure sore such as occurs in an unconscious or paralysed patient.

Communicating

It is important that the patient, and when appropriate the relatives, are educated about pressure sores and their prevention. The preventive and educational process should be a team approach utilising the nurse, physiotherapist, occupational therapist, social worker and the doctor.

Breathing

A patient who has impairment of his cardiovascular system even for a short period of time is at increased risk of developing a pressure sore.

Eating and drinking

The patient's nutritional status should be assessed by the dietician and the appropriate intervention implemented. The nurse may offer the patient high-calorie, high-protein drinks, unless otherwise instructed, as an extra to the diet he is already eating. If the patient is unable to maintain a satisfactory nutritional status by the oral route, nasogastric or parenteral nutrition may be required.

Eliminating

A patient who is incontinent must have his skin kept as free of contamination as possible. Problems of eliminating may be overcome by bladder or bowel training programmes or by treating the underlying cause, e.g. urinary retention with overflow can manifest as urinary incontinence. Following incontinence, the skin should be washed and dried thoroughly without vigorous rubbing, as this can cause maceration of the skin tissue. Soap should be used with caution due to its drying and oil-reducing effects; skin which is dry and lacking in natural oils will break down more readily. A barrier cream may be used, but with caution, as it may interfere with the oxygen and moisture exchange of the skin. Incontinence aids such as a penile sheath or Kylie drawsheet may be of benefit in maintaining a dry environment.

Relevance to the
activities of living
continued

Personal cleansing and dressing

The nurse should use the form of assessment she is familiar with to calculate the patient's risk factor for the development of a pressure sore. A commonly used scale is the Norton scale.

When a patient is confined to bed, the use of a bedcage can greatly reduce the pressure created by the bed linen on the body. Sheets and blankets should be left loose at the edges of the bed. Bed linen should be maintained in a clean, dry and wrinkle-free condition.

As capillary pressure, shearing and friction forces are known to be some of the predisposing factors in the development of a pressure sore, care has to be instituted to reduce these factors. The capillary pressure can be relieved by altering the patient's body position at regular intervals, such as 2-hourly, or more frequently depending on the individual patient's 'at risk' assessment. Shearing and friction forces exerted on the patient's skin tissue can be reduced by utilising a skilled lifting technique when moving him, and positioning of the patient to prevent sliding in any one direction while in bed or in a chair. Adjusting the mattress to maintain the patient's knees in a slightly flexed position while the thighs remain supported, or the use of a padded footboard, can be of help to reduce sliding.

Attention must be paid to the patient's clothing, as buttons, zips, belts and even hard objects like loose change in pockets, have been known to produce a pressure sore.

Controlling body temperature

A patient suffering from hypothermia is more likely to develop a pressure sore due to the effect of the temperature change on the cardiovascular system.

Mobilising

Early ambulation is of great benefit in the prevention of a pressure sore.

A patient who is utilising an aid to mobility is susceptible to the development of a pressure sore at the point of contact of the aid with the body, e.g. a patient who uses a pair of crutches may develop redness of his hands due to the alteration in distribution of body weight. Involuntary muscle movements and joint contracture can interfere with body positioning and can create an increase in shearing and friction forces of the patient's skin tissue.

Working and playing

A pressure sore may increase the patient's hospitalisation period and may have resultant effects on his social status. The nurse must implement care to prevent patient boredom, depression and anxiety about his family's social needs. The social worker may need to be involved in this intervention.

Expressing sexuality

The nurse must provide adequate privacy during the nursing practice. The patient's individual wishes should be observed when possible, which will help to maintain his self-esteem.

Sleeping

Skin care for the prevention and treatment of a pressure sore must be maintained throughout the 24-hour period.

Suggested reading

Crow R 1988 The challenge of pressure sores. Nursing Times 84(38) September 21: 68–73

David J, Chapman R, Chapman E, Lockett B 1983 An investigation of current methods used in nursing for the care of patients with established pressure sores. Nursing Practice Research Unit, Northwick Park Hospital and Clinical Research Centre, Harrow, Middlesex

Dawes H, Small D, Glen E 1990 Adding computers to the armoury (describes computerised history-taking and assessment of incontinent patients). Nursing Times 86(46) November 14: 68–69

Horne E 1986 How safe is sunbathing? Professional Nurse 1(10) July: 268–269

Irvine L 1988 Incontinence in the young woman. Senior Nurse 8(3) March: 16–18

Kennedy J 1989 Ring cushions – an outmoded treatment. Nursing Times 85(48) November 29: 34–35

Macaulay M, Henry G 1990 Drop in and do well (discusses establishment of a continence clinic). Nursing Times 86(46) November 14: 65–66

McSweeney P 1989 Continence: prevent, retrain, treat, contain. Nursing Times 85(46) November 15: 68–69

Mowlam V, North K, Myers C 1986 Managing faecal incontinence. Nursing Times 82(48) November 26: 55–59

Roper N, Logan W, Tierney A 1990 The elements of nursing, 3rd edn. Churchill Livingstone, Edinburgh, pp 218–225

Spenceley P 1988 Norton v Waterlow. Nursing Times 84(32) August 10: 52–53

Waterlow J 1985 A risk assessment card. Nursing Times 81(48) November 27: 49–55

Walsh M, Ford P 1989 Nursing rituals – research and rational actions. Heinemann Nursing, Oxford, ch 7

There are two parts to this section:

1 Washing of the hair
2 Care of the infested head

The concluding subsection, 'Relevance to the activities of living', refers to the two practices collectively.

Objectives

By the end of this section you should know how to:

- prepare the patient for these nursing practices

- carry out washing of the hair and care of the infested head

- collect and prepare the equipment

Related information

Revision of the anatomy and physiology of the skin with special reference to the hair follicles of the scalp.

Revision of the life cycle of the head louse (pediculus capitis).

Review of the health authority policy on the use and type of insecticide.

1 WASHING OF THE HAIR

Some indications for washing of the hair

The hair covers the skin of the scalp, therefore sweat, sebum, dust and dead epithelial cells become trapped between the hair strands. The patient's hair, if left unwashed, may appear greasy and limp, and generally makes him feel unkempt. The patient may be unable to maintain his hair hygiene due to the effect of disease or injury or following surgery, or because of age (either a young child or a frail elderly person).

Equipment

Basin
Large container of warm water   } for a bedfast patient
Container for used water
Small jug or hair spray tap attachment
Cotton towels
Polythene sheeting
Patient's shampoo
Patient's own comb and/or brush
Disposable paper towel
Disposable plastic apron
Hair dryer
Trolley for equipment
Receptacle for soiled disposables

Guidelines for this nursing practice

- explain the nursing practice to the patient and gain his consent and cooperation
- collect and prepare the equipment
- wash the hands

Bedfast patient

- help the patient into a comfortable position, e.g. patient's head overhanging the edge of the bed
- protect the patient's clothing, pillows and bedclothes using the polythene sheeting
- place a towel around the patient's shoulders
- position the basin under the patient's head
- protect the patient's eyes
- using the basin to catch the water, wet the hair
- apply the shampoo

Ambulant patient

- help the patient to the bathroom and ensure that he is sitting comfortably
- protect his clothing using the polythene sheeting
- drape a towel around his shoulders
- protect the patient's eyes
- using the small jug or the hair spray tap attachment, wet the hair and apply the shampoo
- rinse off the lather and repeat if the patient wishes

- ensure the patient's privacy
- observe the patient throughout this activity

- rinse off the lather and repeat if the patient wishes
- towel the hair dry
- assist the patient to comb his hair into the usual style and dry using the hair dryer
- ensure that the patient is left feeling as comfortable as possible
- dispose of the equipment safely
- document the nursing practice appropriately, monitor after-effects and report abnormal findings immediately

- towel the hair dry
- assist the patient to comb his hair into his usual style and dry using the hair dryer
- ensure the patient is left feeling as comfortable as possible
- dispose of the equipment safely
- document the nursing practice appropriately, monitor after-effects and report abnormal findings immediately

A patient can also have his hair washed during a shower or an immersion bath, using a hair spray tap attachment.

2   CARE OF THE INFESTED HEAD

Some indications for care of the infested head

Scalp infestation is the parasitic infestation of the scalp by the head louse. The louse and its pre-louse stage, the nit, cause irritation which may lead to scratching and potential infection of the abrasions. An insecticide is used:

- to remove the parasite
- to prevent the infestation from spreading to family members, other patients and staff

Equipment

Insecticide can be used in shampoo or lotion form

Medicated shampoo treatment

Shampoo containing carbaryl or malathion
Disposable cap and gown
Fine-tooth comb
Equipment as for hair washing (see p. 262)

Medicated lotion treatment

Head lotion containing carbaryl or malathion
Polythene sheeting
Disposable paper towel, cap and gown
Fine-tooth comb

12 hours later, equipment for hair washing (see p. 262)

Trolley or tray for equipment
Receptacle for soiled disposables

Guidelines for this nursing practice

- explain the nursing practice to the patient and gain his consent and cooperation, and explain that you will wear a cap and gown
- collect and prepare the equipment
- wash the hands
- apply a disposable cap and gown for personal protection
- ensure the patient's privacy
- observe the patient throughout this activity
- assist the patient into a comfortable position

Medicated shampoo method

- follow the Guidelines as for washing the hair
- protect the patient's eyes
- use the medicated shampoo as recommended by the manufacturer
- rinse the hair thoroughly
- comb the hair with the fine-tooth comb, collecting the nits and lice on a disposable paper towel with each stroke of the comb
- allow the patient's hair to dry
- ensure the patient is left feeling as comfortable as possible
- disinfect the patient's comb and/or hairbrush using the shampoo
- dispose of the equipment safely
- remove the protective cap and gown and dispose of them safely
- document the nursing practice appropriately, monitor after-effects and report abnormal findings immediately

Medicated head lotion method

- protect the patient's clothing using the polythene sheeting
- protect the patient's eyes
- apply the head lotion as recommended by the manufacturer, paying particular attention to the area above the ears and the nape of the neck
- leave the hair to dry naturally
- disinfect the patient's comb and/or hairbrush
- 12 hours later, wash the hair with a normal shampoo
- comb the hair with the fine-tooth comb, collecting the nits and lice on a disposable paper towel with each stroke of the comb
- allow the patient's hair to dry naturally
- ensure the patient is left feeling as comfortable as possible
- disinfect the fine-tooth comb with the head lotion
- dispose of the equipment safely
- remove the cap and gown and dispose of them safely
- document the nursing practice appropriately, monitor after-effects and report abnormal findings immediately

Either of the two forms of treatment should be repeated as recommended by the manufacturer, and according to the success of the treatment.

Hair Care

Relevance to the activities of living

Maintaining a safe environment

Although hair care does not require aseptic technique, all equipment should be clean or disposable and all precautions be taken to prevent cross-infection. The nurse should wash her hands before commencing and on completion of hair care.

The nurse should test the temperature of the water prior to washing a patient's hair and be aware of any temperature change during the nursing practice, so that the patient's comfort is being maintained. Protecting the patient's eyes reduces the potential problem of accidental introduction of shampoo or the medicated head lotion into the eyes; they would act as irritants to the eyes. Once the infestation is noted, treatment should start immediately as the condition spreads rapidly. Transmission of the louse is by direct physical contact or by contact with an infested comb, hairbrush, wig, hat or bedding. All family members and close contacts must be treated at the same time as the patient, otherwise re-infestation of the patient will occur. For her own safety, the nurse may wear a disposable cap and gown during the treatment of an infested scalp.

If left untreated, the sufferer may develop any of a variety of complications such as impetigo, dermatitis or undefined general malaise.

The louse can develop resistance to an insecticide. The suggested insecticides are the two in common use at present, but advice from the pharmacy department should be sought about the current recommended insecticide.

Communicating

The patient with an infested scalp must be given a tactful, easily understood explanation about the reason and the form of treatment. The patient's relatives and/or close contacts will also need to be informed about the infestation and given the necessary information about their own treatment. Some education of the patient and his family about the head louse may be necessary.

Personal cleansing and dressing

For normal hair cleanliness, the use of a dry shampoo can be of benefit to the patient who is unable to have his hair washed using shampoo and water.

As far as the infested head is concerned, the nits remain firmly attached to the hair even following insecticide treatment, therefore the fine-tooth comb must be used to remove them. The patient's hair should be left to dry naturally after insecticide application, as most of the lotions have an inflammable alcoholic base.

Expressing sexuality

A patient's hair should be kept in good condition as this helps to create a positive body image and maintain his self-esteem.

The nurse should style the patient's hair in the usual manner or as the patient wishes, as this helps to maintain his individuality.

Most people are embarrassed if it is discovered that the hair is infested with lice, and although the nurse should wear a disposable cap and gown while assisting the patient to remove the infestation, the explanation for doing so should be tactful and should not detract from the patient's dignity and self-esteem.

Suggested reading   Brunner L, Suddarth D 1988 Textbook of medical–surgical nursing. J. B. Lippincott, Philadelphia, p 1290
Butler M 1981 Infestation. Nursing 1(23) March: 988–990
Cluroe S 1990 How to deal with head lice. Nursing 4(16) August 9: 9–12
De-Mont A 1985 Don't let your hair down. Nursing Times Community Outlook 81(37) September 11: 16–17 (Products available for treatment of head lice and dandruff)
Mohylnycky N 1983 Parasitic skin infections. Nursing 2(9) January: 246–248
Roberts C 1989 Head lice. Practice Nurse 2(3) July: 108–111
Roper N, Logan W, Tierney A 1990 The elements of nursing, 3rd edn. Churchill Livingstone, Edinburgh, pp 203, 209–217

Mouth Care

Objectives

By the end of this section you should know how to:

- prepare the patient for this nursing practice
- collect and prepare the equipment
- carry out mouth care according to the individual needs of the patient

Related information

Revision of the anatomy and physiology of the mouth, with special reference to the teeth, the salivary glands and the oral mucosa.

Revision of pharmaceutical literature related to mouthwashes and mouth-cleaning preparations in current use.

Review of health authority policy related to mouth care.

Some indications for mouth care

Mouth care is the use of a toothbrush and paste, a mouthwash or other mouth-cleaning preparation to help the patient maintain the cleanliness of his teeth or dentures, and to encourage the flow of saliva to maintain a healthy oropharyngeal mucosa. This nursing practice is also known as oral hygiene and may be required:

- for any patient who has not eaten for a period of time or whose diet is restricted, e.g. during the preoperative or postoperative period, and especially for patients following oral or abdominal surgery
- for patients who are dehydrated for any reason
- for patients suffering from nausea or vomiting
- for patients being treated with oxygen therapy which has a drying effect on the oral mucosa
- for patients who are having radiotherapy or cytotoxic medication for malignant disease, as this may affect the cells of the oral mucosa

The frequency of mouth care will vary for each individual. Intensive mouth care may be carried out every 2 hours, whereas mouthwashes may only be required 2 or 3 times a day.

Equipment

Suitable tray or trolley
Pencil torch
Spatula
Toothbrush
Toothpaste
Container for dentures (appropriately labelled)
Beaker
Bowl or receiver
Towel or other protective covering
Mouthwash solution
Receptacle for disposables

Additional equipment for specialised mouth care as required

Mouth care pack or equivalent equipment
Plastic gloves (non-sterile)
Foam sticks
Cotton buds
Prescribed medication eg: antifungal agent, if thrush is diagnosed
Solution for mouth cleaning
Lubrication for lips, e.g. Vaseline
Suction equipment

Toothbrush and toothpaste

The patient's own equipment may be used if available, otherwise a soft nylon brush and toothpaste can be supplied. Usually this is the most appropriate equipment for this nursing practice.

Solutions for mouthwashes

Various solutions are available. Local practice or individual prescription will influence the choice of preparation used.

All solutions used should be clearly labelled and diluted according to instructions. The procedure for checking the preparation is as for administration of medications (p. 12).

Saline: This can be made up using common salt, one level teaspoon (4.5 g approx) made up in 500 ml water. It is also available in sterile sachets. This is an effective mouthwash for patients who have had oral surgery, especially dental extractions.

Thymol: This is prepared in solution with glycerin and is the main component of most mouthwash tablets. It has a mild antiseptic effect and is well tolerated when diluted to suit the patient's taste.

Sodium bicarbonate: This may be made up immediately prior to use. One level teaspoon of powder in 500 ml of water is a useful mouthwash for dissolving mucus and debris. A stronger solution can be used for soaking dentures before cleaning them.

Corsodyl: This is a commercial preparation containing chlorhexidine which is thought to inhibit plaque formation. It may be prescribed for patients having cytotoxic therapy.

Cold water: This may be the most refreshing and appropriate mouthwash to use after brushing the teeth.

Equipment
continued

Other aids for mouth care (if permitted)

Soda water: This may be appreciated as an alternative mouth wash.

Ice cubes: These may be sucked, but the number should be limited, if the patient has restricted oral intake.

Fresh fruit: This can be sucked and removed. Pineapple, if allowed, can be very refreshing and will stimulate saliva.

Solutions for mouth cleaning

Any mouthwash solution can be used for mouth cleaning, as well as solutions which actively stimulate the flow of saliva.

A mild toothpaste applied with a soft toothbrush remains the most efficient method of mouth cleaning.

The toothbrush may be dipped in any mouthwash/mouth cleaning solution acceptable to the patient.

Mouth-care pack

This prepared sterile pack is used when intensive mouth care is needed for patients for whom a mouthwash alone, or tooth-brushing, is not appropriate. The pack may contain:
— plastic tray divided into compartments to hold the mouth-cleaning solution
— plastic forceps
— dental rolls
— gauze swabs

If the pack is not available a sterile mouth-care tray can be assembled using:
— foil tray
— gallipot
— plastic forceps
— gauze swabs
— dental rolls

The mouth-care pack should be covered, labelled with the patient's name, the date, cleaned and replenished after use, and replaced every 24 hours or as required.

Guidelines for this nursing practice

- explain the nursing practice and gain the patient's consent and cooperation

- collect and prepare the equipment

- ensure the patient's privacy

- help the patient into a comfortable sitting position, either in bed or on a chair

- place some protective material over the patient's chest and under his chin. The patient's own towel could be used

- observe the patient throughout this activity

- don clean plastic gloves if required

- ask or help the patient to remove his dentures and place them in a labelled bowl of clean water

- examine the patient's mouth and tongue using the torch and spatula, and observe the condition of the teeth, gums and mucosa. Note any ulcers or sores and the condition of the lips

- discuss with the patient, if possible, the most suitable and acceptable mouth care for his particular needs

- help the patient to clean his teeth or his dentures with his toothbrush and toothpaste

- offer a suitable mouthwash, explaining that it should not be swallowed, and help to hold the equipment as necessary

- offer tissues for drying the mouth

- help to apply lubrication to the lips as required. This can be done by placing the lubricant on a gloved finger and applying it directly, or using a dental roll or a gauze swab, or the patient may apply it himself

- return the patient's clean dentures to him in a bowl of clean water and encourage him to wear them

- ensure the patient is left feeling as comfortable as possible

- dispose of equipment safely

- document the nursing practice appropriately and report any deterioration or improvement in the condition of the mouth, as well as abnormal findings, immediately

Mouth Care

Guidelines for this
nursing practice
continued

Intensive mouth care for dependent patients

- explain the nursing practice and gain the patient's consent and cooperation if possible

- ensure the patient's privacy

- help the patient into a comfortable position

- collect and prepare the equipment including the mouth cleaning pack or tray

- don clean plastic gloves

- remove dentures if present

- examine the patient's mouth as before

- clean all round the mouth, gums and tongue with the mouth-cleaning solution, using a soft toothbrush if possible. A gauze swab wrapped carefully round a gloved finger and dipped into the solution may be used, but it depends on the patient's cooperation (Fig. 6.5). A gauze swab wrapped round a pair of plastic forceps, or a dental roll held lengthways in forceps or fingers, can also be used. In some instances a foam stick may be suitable.

- help the patient to use a mouthwash if possible, or rinse the mouth with a gauze swab soaked in mouthwash solution allowing the patient to suck it.

- help the patient to clean his dentures or clean them for him using toothbrush and toothpaste under a running tap if possible

- proceed with the nursing practice as before

Figure 6.5
Using a covered finger to cleanse the mouth

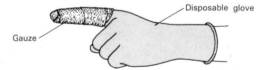

Mouth care for an unconscious patient

Mouth care guidelines as for a dependent patient, except for the following:

- position the patient on his side, with no pillow, and his head supported so that no secretion or mouth-cleaning solution can flow into the trachea and be inhaled

- place waterproof material on the bed before placing tissues under the lower side of the face to absorb solution and saliva draining from the mouth

- check that suction equipment is at hand and in working order, and if required, perform oral suction before commencing the nursing practice

The dentures should have been removed, cleaned, appropriately labelled and stored with the patient's belongings on admission (see Care of the unconscious patient, p. 312).

Maintaining a safe environment

The oral mucosa itself is part of the body's defence against infection. Mouth care which helps to keep the teeth and oral mucosa in good condition is important in maintaining a safe environment for the patient.

Although mouth care does not need aseptic technique, all the equipment should be clean or disposable, and all precautions should be taken to prevent any cross-infection. The nurse should wash her hands before commencing and on completion of mouth care for each patient.

The nurse herself should be protected from any blood-borne viral infection which might be present in the saliva, e.g. hepatitis B or HIV. As a precaution it is advisable for gloves to be worn for all mouth care which might involve direct contact with the oral mucosa or oral secretions.

Patients who are having cytotoxic medication for malignant disease, e.g. leukaemia, may be at greater risk of infection than normal. The treatment itself may also affect the cells of the oral mucosa. A special mouth care regimen may be prescribed for these patients using mouthwashes, suspensions or creams. If possible the patients themselves should apply these once the nurse has shown the procedure, to minimise the risk of cross-infection. The importance of this care in the prevention of infection should be explained to the patient, and the nurse may use this time as an opportunity for patient education.

Mouthwashes should only be given to patients who are alert and well orientated, with a good cough reflex, otherwise there is a danger of accidental inhalation of the solution.

Communicating

A patient who has a dry or infected mouth will find it uncomfortable to talk, and dry lips can also be painful when speaking, so appropriate mouth care can help with communication. Having a mouth which feels fresh can help to raise the patient's morale, and encourage him to take an interest in other people and his surroundings.

Breathing

Patients who have a cough and sputum may appreciate regular mouthwashes to clear mucus which may have lodged round the teeth and gums. A mouthwash should be given after chest physiotherapy to freshen the mouth and encourage a feeling of well-being, although an opportunity to clean the teeth may be even more welcome.

Mouth Care

Relevance to the
activities of living
continued

Eating and drinking

The opportunity for mouth care should be provided for all patients after meals. They should be encouraged to clean teeth and/or dentures, as well as to rinse the mouth. This may require the nurse to assemble the equipment and give appropriate help. This regular encouragement should form part of patient education in personal hygiene. The importance of a healthy mouth, teeth and gums should be emphasised.

A dry or 'dirty' mouth may discourage a patient from eating. Good mouth care can be a help in promoting the appetite and be an encouragement to eat, when this is important to aid recovery.

Conversely, patients who are not allowed to eat by the oral route will need frequent mouth care to maintain a healthy mucosa.

An adequate fluid intake is an additional help in maintaining a moist, healthy oral environment.

Personal cleansing and dressing

An important part of this activity of living is the patient's own oral hygiene. The nurse should be able to identify any associated problems during her assessment of the patient, and this may be an opportunity for patient education in relation to dental and oral hygiene.

Using a toothbrush effectively: Brushing the teeth loosens and removes debris trapped in the spaces and also prevents the growth of plaque, which harbours bacteria and may be a precursor of dental caries. The brushing also stimulates the blood circulation in the gums and helps to keep the soft tissue healthy. The teeth should be brushed firmly with strokes directed away from the gums; upward strokes for the lower teeth, and downward strokes for the upper teeth. The teeth should not be brushed from side to side or up and down, or debris will be redeposited in the spaces between the teeth, or along the edge of the gums. Inner aspects of the teeth should be brushed in the same way. Efficient tooth cleaning should not be hurried. The mouth should be well rinsed several times during and after tooth cleaning. Facilities for cleaning the teeth or dentures should be offered after meals for all patients who are not self-caring.

The correct use of dental floss can be included when discussing dental hygiene.

The importance of regular visits to the dentist should also be emphasised when the opportunity arises.

Expressing sexuality

Sexuality can be expressed positively in the form of non-verbal communication. As an example, smiling is an important facet of this, and is used as a way of projecting self to other people; teeth and gums which are well cared for enhance the body image and the feeling of well-being. If a patient is feeling depressed, appropriate mouth care and a fresh mouthwash may encourage a male patient to agree to having a shave in preparation for meeting his visitors, and a female patient may feel encouraged to put on make-up, lipstick and perfume.

Suggested reading   Auld E M 1988 Oral health. Geriatric Nursing 9(6) November/December: 340–341
Harrison A 1987 Denture care. Nursing Times 83(19) May 13: 28–29
McCord F, Stalker A 1988 Brushing up on oral care. Nursing Times 84(13) March 30:
40–41
Miller R et al 1987 Oral health care for hospitalised patients. Journal of Nurse
Education 26(9) November: 362–366
Roper N, Logan W, Tierney A 1990 The elements of nursing, 3rd edn. Churchill
Livingstone, Edinburgh, pp 202–229
Shepherd G et al 1987 The mouth trap. Nursing Times 83(19) May13: 25–27
Thompson J 1990 Oral hygiene and dental care. Community Outlook. January: 10–15
Walsh M, Ford P 1989 Nursing rituals – research and rational actions. Heinemann
Nursing, Oxford, pp 112–114, 154–156
Watson R 1989 Care of the mouth. Nursing 3(46) October 26: 20–24

Controlling Body Temperature

Body Temperature

Objectives

By the end of this section you should know how to:

- prepare the patient for this nursing practice
- collect and prepare the equipment
- measure and record the body temperature at the axilla, in the oral cavity and in the rectum

Related information

Revision of the anatomy and physiology of the skin in relation to the control of body temperature and of the temperature-regulating centre, and related body mechanisms associated with heat production and heat loss.

Revision of the anatomy of the area where the temperature is to be measured.

Some indications for recording body temperature

A temperature recording is a measurement of body temperature in degrees Celsius (°C) using a calibrated clinical thermometer or an electronic probe. The axilla, the oral cavity or the rectum are the sites which may be chosen for the recording. For each patient the site chosen for measuring the temperature should be used consistently, so that any changes in temperature can be monitored. The normal range of body temperature is between 36–37.5°C. The upper and lower limits of survival are not known exactly, but are thought to be at body temperatures of 45°C and 25°C respectively (Fig. 7.1).

The recording of body temperature may be required:

- to establish a baseline temperature, e.g. when patients are admitted to hospital or clinic

- to monitor fluctuations in temperature, e.g. for patients during the postoperative period, temperature fluctuations can indicate developing infection or the presence of a deep venous thrombosis

- to monitor signs of incompatibility when patients are receiving a blood transfusion

- to monitor the temperature of patients being treated for an infection

- to monitor the temperature of patients recovering from hypothermia

Figure 7.1
Range of normal/abnormal body temperature (oral) (Reproduced with permission from Roper N, Logan W, Tierney A 1990 The elements of nursing, 3rd edn. Churchill Livingstone, Edinburgh)

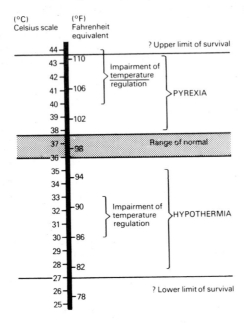

The frequency of the recording will depend on the reason for monitoring body temperature, and on the patient's condition.

Equipment

Tray

Appropriate thermometer, e.g.
— clinical thermometer
— disposable thermometer
— electronic thermometer plus probe

Alcohol-impregnated swabs, e.g. Mediswabs

Watch with a seconds hand

Tissues

Receptacle for disposables

Additional equipment as required:

Disposable sleeve for clinical thermometer, e.g. Steritemp sleeve

Disposable probe cover for electronic probe

Lubricant for rectal thermometer, e.g. petroleum jelly

Clinical thermometers

These thermometers have a glass bulb filled with mercury which expands along a calibrated glass tube in response to contact with the warmer temperature of human body tissues. The tube has a constriction above the bulb to prevent the mercury from returning to its original position when removed from the site of the recording, thus allowing the temperature measurement to be accurately read. Before commencing a recording, the mercury in the tube should be shaken down to give a reading level with the lowest calibrated figure on the thermometer. The clinical thermometer should remain in position for at least 4 minutes to prevent a false low result. Research has shown that thermometers should be in situ for 4–9 minutes (see Suggested reading).

There are various types of clinical thermometer (Fig. 7.2):

Oral/axillary thermometer. This is used for measuring the oral or axillary temperature. It has an oval-shaped clear glass-covered mercury bulb and is calibrated between 35°C and 43.5°C.

Rectal thermometer. This is used for measuring the rectal temperature. It has a blue-coloured, more rounded mercury bulb and is calibrated between 35°C and 43.5°C.

Low reading thermometer. This is specially calibrated to record readings of temperature between 25°C and 40°C and is used to record the temperature of patients suffering from hypothermia.

Figure 7.2
Clinical glass thermometers
A Oral/axillary
B Rectal
C Low reading

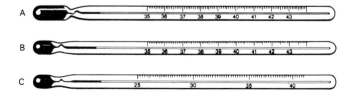

Equipment
continued

Disposable thermometers

These have rapid-reacting heat-sensitive chemicals in the recording head, so that a recording can be made in 60 seconds. They are used for oral recording and are discarded after one use. Similar equipment is available for measuring skin temperature.

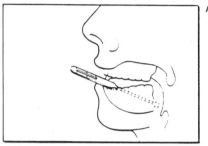

A Thermometer in situ

Figure 7.3
Disposable thermometer with rechargeable, battery-operated readout unit

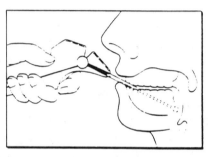

B Recording the oral body temperature with readout unit

Electronic thermometers

These have probes which must be protected by disposable covers before being placed at the recording site. They are connected to equipment which gives an electronic readout of the temperature in 25–35 seconds. Various types of electronic temperature-recording equipment are available (Fig. 7.4). Some probes are designed especially for oral or axillary temperatures, and others for rectal recordings (refer to manufacturer's instructions).

Figure 7.4
Example of an electronic thermometer

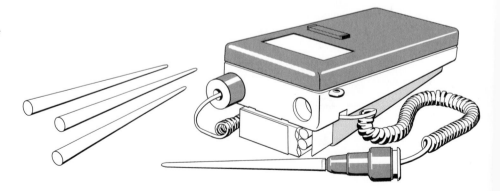

Guidelines for this nursing practice

Guidelines are given for temperature recording in three sites using a clinical thermometer, but the principles can be adapted for any type of thermometer.

Axilla

- explain the nursing practice and gain the patient's consent and cooperation. Ensure that he has not recently had a hot bath or been engaged in strenuous exercise
- ensure the patient's privacy
- help the patient into a comfortable position with the back and shoulders well supported, so that he may remain in that position for a few minutes. He may be either sitting or lying
- help the patient to remove or adjust his clothing to expose one axilla
- observe the patient throughout this activity
- dry the skin of the axilla by wiping with a tissue. A film of moisture between the skin area and the thermometer bulb can cause an inaccurate reading
- check the thermometer reading and shake the thermometer to return the mercury column to 35°C
- clean the thermometer by wiping it with an alcohol solution (e.g. Mediswab) and allow the alcohol solution to evaporate
- place the bulb end of the thermometer in the axilla where the skin surfaces will surround it

- help the patient to hold his arm across his chest to retain the thermometer in the correct position
- leave the thermometer in position for the required time to allow the maximum temperature to be measured – a minimum of 4 minutes
- remain with the patient if required
- remove the thermometer
- read the temperature measured by the thermometer
- wipe the thermometer with alcohol solution
- shake the thermometer to return the mercury to the bulb, and a reading of 35°C on the thermometer
- ensure the patient is left feeling as comfortable as possible
- dispose of equipment safely
- document the temperature reading in the patient's records, compare the reading with previous recordings and report abnormal findings immediately

Guidelines for this
nursing practice
continued

Oral cavity

- explain the nursing practice and gain the patient's consent and cooperation. Ensure that he has not recently had a hot or cold drink, or a hot bath, or been engaged in strenuous exercise

- help the patient into a comfortable position

- prepare the thermometer as for an axillary temperature recording

- apply a disposable sleeve if required

- place the thermometer under the patient's tongue so that the bulb lies adjacent to the frenulum at the junction of the floor of the mouth and the base of the tongue, on either the right or left side. A maximum temperature recording will be obtained from one of these two 'heat pockets' in the mouth (Fig. 7.5)

- explain to the patient the importance of closing only the lips round the thermometer, and not biting it, so that oral temperature is maintained

- leave the thermometer in position for the required time

- remove the thermometer and proceed as for an axillary temperature recording

Figure 7.5
Oral cavity
A Position of heat pocket on mouth floor
B Thermometer in position in a heat pocket (Reproduced with permission from Roper N, Logan W, Tierney A 1990 The elements of nursing, 3rd edn. Churchill Livingstone, Edinburgh)

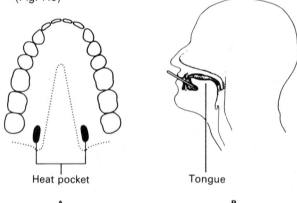

Heat pocket   Tongue

A   B

Rectum

- explain the nursing practice to the patient and gain his consent and cooperation

- ensure the patient's privacy

- help the patient into a comfortable position lying on his side with knees bent

- prepare the thermometer as for an axillary temperature recording

- apply a disposable sleeve

- lubricate the protected end of the thermometer

- gently insert the thermometer into the patient's anus for 2–4 cm and hold the thermometer in position for the required time

- remove the thermometer, dispose of the protective sleeve and proceed as for an axillary temperature recording

Relevance to the activities of living

Maintaining a safe environment

Temperature recording is a non-invasive practice; however, the nurse should wash her hands before and after the recording to prevent any cross-infection. The equipment should be kept clean and rectal thermometers should be stored separately from other thermometers. Clinical thermometers should be handled and stored with care; broken glass and mercury vapour can both cause harm to patients and staff.

Oral temperature recording should only be used for adult patients who are alert, well orientated and able to cooperate in carrying out the procedure.

Rectal temperature recordings should be used for infants. Children and all adults who are unable to cooperate, e.g. due to breathlessness, confusion or unconsciousness, should have an axilla or rectal temperature recorded. Electronic probes are more suitable and less traumatic than clinical thermometers for recording a rectal temperature, and are being used increasingly.

The probe or bulb of a rectal thermometer should be covered by a disposable cover or sleeve before lubrication and insertion. This not only prevents cross-infection, but also prevents any damage to the surrounding mucosa. When no specialised cover is available, the probe can be inserted into the finger of a plastic glove before insertion, the rest of the glove remaining outside the body, and easily removable.

In a general ward, fans should not be used to cool patients who have a pyrexia caused by infection. The increased movement of air may increase the risk of cross-infection in the area.

Communicating

While the oral temperature is being recorded the patient should not speak. Apart from the danger of breaking the thermometer the passage of air through the mouth while talking affects the temperature reading, and this should be explained to the patient.

Eating and drinking

Patients with a raised body temperature are prescribed an increased fluid intake to compensate for the increased loss of fluid due to perspiration. Fluid intake should be encouraged and accurately recorded. Fluid balance charts should be maintained for all patients with a pyrexia, to monitor hydration.

Eliminating

Fluid output should be recorded, and fluid balance charts accurately maintained for all patients with other than normal body temperature.

Pyrexia may result in decreased output of urine, which may be concentrated and dark in colour. This may be a result of dehydration due to increased fluid loss from perspiration.

Body Temperature

Relevance to the
activities of living
continued

Personal cleansing and dressing

Clothing may have to be adjusted for the recording of both axillary and rectal temperatures. The nurse should gain the patient's help and cooperation during this nursing practice.

The amount of clothing and bed covers may be adjusted depending on the patient's reaction to a change of body temperature. A patient with a pyrexia may feel very warm or very cold.

Occasionally the patient may be sponged with tepid water to try to reduce a raised body temperature. It may be prescribed for patients who have damage to the temperature-controlling centre in the hypothalamus, causing hyperpyrexia (see Tepid sponging, p. 286).

A bed bath should be given as frequently as required to ensure the patient's comfort, as patients with a raised body temperature perspire profusely.

Patients with a pyrexia may become dehydrated due to excess insensible fluid loss. Frequent mouth care should be given to maintain a healthy mucosa, and to help alleviate the 'dry mouth' effect associated with pyrexia.

Controlling body temperature

Any change in body temperature may indicate the patient's response to an adverse environment. Under normal conditions the body's internal temperature remains remarkably constant at around 37°C. The range of normal recordings in the adult is 36–37.5°C (see Fig. 7.1). Children have a correspondingly higher range of body temperature than adults due to their increased metabolic rate.

For a healthy person the axillary temperature is at the lower range of normal; the rectal temperature is at the upper range of normal, and the oral temperature somewhere in between. For each patient the site chosen for the temperature recording should be used consistently to enable changes in body temperature to be accurately monitored.

Both a core temperature and a peripheral temperature may be recorded for seriously ill patients suffering from, for example, cardiogenic, bacteraemic or haemorrhagic shock. Under normal conditions, there should not be more than 3°C difference between the core temperature and the peripheral temperature.

The *core temperature* should be recorded at a site where the reading will be as near as possible to the temperature of the blood. An electronic probe may be inserted into the rectum or the oesophagus, and attached to an electronic monitor to give a continuous core temperature reading.

The *peripheral temperature* may be recorded by a small flat probe taped to the patient's big toe to give a continuous read-out of the peripheral temperature on the electronic monitor.

Pyrexia is the term given to a rise in body temperature above 37.5°C, and this should be reported.

Hyperpyrexia is the term given to a rise in body temperature above 40°C. Body temperature above 41°C or prolonged hyperpyrexia may cause damage to brain cell function and result in associated fits or rigors. Any hyperpyrexia should be treated as an emergency and reported immediately.

Hypothermia is the term given to a fall in body temperature below 35°C. Warming a patient suffering from hypothermia should be done gradually (a rise of 0.5°C per hour is suggested) under medical guidance. Sudden heating of the periphery of the body can divert the blood from the vital centres and cause further shock.

Expressing sexuality

The recording of a rectal temperature can be an uncomfortable and undignified procedure. The reason for this choice of site should be explained to the patient. A nurse who has good communication skills can help to maintain the patient's dignity.

Sleeping

When an electronic thermometer is in situ, there is no need to disturb a patient who is sleeping. When other types of thermometer are used, it requires clinical judgement to decide whether or not to waken a patient, especially during the night, in order to record his temperature.

Suggested reading

Baker N et al 1984 The effect of type of thermometer and length of time inserted on oral temperature recordings of afebrile subjects. Nursing Research 33(2) March/April: 109–111

Burke N L 1988 Inadvertent hypothermia. Journal of Gerontological Nursing 14(6) June 26: 36–71

Closs J 1987 Oral temperature measurement. Nursing Times 83(1) January 7: 36–39

Heidenreich T, Guiffre M 1990 Postoperative temperature measurement. Nursing Research 39(3) May/June: 153–155

Hillman H 1987 The cold that kills. Nursing Times 83(1) January 7: 19–20

Neff J et al 1989 Effect of respiratory patterns on sublingual temperature. Research in Nursing & Health 12(3) June: 195–202

Robichaud E, Esktrand E et al 1989 Comparison of electronic and glass thermometers. Canadian Journal of Nursing Research 21(1) Spring: 61–73

Roper N, Logan W, Tierney A 1990 The elements of nursing, 3rd edn. Churchill Livingstone, Edinburgh, pp 230–243

Walsh M, Ford P 1989 Nursing rituals – research and rational actions. Heinemann Nursing, Oxford pp 50–53

Tepid Sponging

Objectives

By the end of this section you should know how to:

- prepare the patient for this nursing practice
- carry out tepid sponging
- collect and prepare the equipment

Related information

Revision of the anatomy and physiology of the skin with special reference to the role of the skin in the maintenance of body temperature.

Revision of temperature recording (see p. 278), bed bathing (see p. 250) and mouth care (see p. 268)

Some indications for tepid sponging

Tepid sponging is the application of water to a patient's skin surface to promote the dispersal of body heat when the body temperature is 39.5°C and over, by utilising the principles of evaporation and conduction.

A patient may show the manifestation of pyrexia when there is:

- invasion by pathogenic microorganisms
- a metabolic disorder
- disease of the nervous system
- malignant/neoplastic disease

Equipment

Equipment for temperature recording (see p. 278)
Equipment for mouth care (see p. 268)
Basin of warm water (30–33°C)
Lotion thermometer
Bowl of ice-cold water for cold compress
Six disposable face cloths or similar items
Three bath towels
Pyjamas or gown
Bed linen
Trolley for equipment
Receptacle for soiled disposables
Receptacle for soiled pyjamas or gown if it belongs to the patient
Receptacle for soiled bed linen

Guidelines for this nursing practice

- explain the nursing practice to the patient and gain his consent and cooperation
- wash the hands
- collect and prepare the equipment required
- ensure the patient's privacy
- observe the patient throughout this activity
- help the patient into a comfortable position
- assess and record the patient's body temperature
- remove excess bed linen and bed appliances if in use, but leave the patient covered with a bed sheet
- help the patient to remove the pyjamas or gown
- place a cold compress to the patient's forehead, axillae and groin area. Renew the compresses as they become warm
- check the temperature of the basin of water using the lotion thermometer
- without using friction, slowly sponge the patient's body with a wet face cloth as suggested in bathing in bed (see p. 250)
- gently pat the patient's skin dry, if required. It is preferable to leave the water to evaporate
- change the face cloths as they become warm, immerse them in the ice-cold water and replace them with cold face cloths
- change all bed linen
- help the patient to dress in pyjamas or gown
- remake the patient's bed
- assess and record the patient's body temperature
- help the patient with mouth care if wished
- ensure that the patient is left feeling as comfortable as possible
- dispose of the equipment safely
- document the nursing practice appropriately, monitor after-effects and report abnormal findings immediately

Tepid Sponging

Relevance to the activities of living

Maintaining a safe environment

Although tepid sponging does not require aseptic technique, all equipment should be clean or disposable and all precautions be taken to prevent cross-infection. The nurse should wash her hands before commencing and on completion of the nursing practice.

The patient should be observed throughout the nursing practice for any sign of an adverse reaction such as shivering and/or an increase in respiration rate. If these arise the nurse must stop the tepid sponge, cover the patient with a blanket and report the adverse reaction immediately.

Disorientation to time can be caused by pyrexia therefore the nurse may need to assist the patient with actual or potential problems as they are identified.

Communicating

The patient may suffer from irritability and anxiety due to the effect of the pyrexia, and the nurse should assist the patient to reduce these problems by attending promptly to his needs. The patient's relatives may require an explanation from the nurse as to the reason for the patient's anxiety and irritability.

Eating and drinking

Following a tepid sponge the patient may be offered a cool drink. It may help him to feel cooler but it also assists in the prevention of dehydration and reduces the discomfort felt by the patient due to a dry mouth. As the patient's metabolic rate is increased during pyrexia, drinks containing protein and carbohydrate are of benefit.

Personal cleansing and dressing

A patient who requires a tepid sponge is, in most circumstances, perspiring freely. It enhances patient comfort if the clothing being worn is made from a non-synthetic fabric such as cotton, as this has a high moisture absorption rate.

The patient's clothing and bed linen should be changed as they become damp with perspiration.

Controlling body temperature

A patient whose body temperature is 39.5°C and above has the actual problem of impairment to the temperature-regulating mechanisms within the body. Tepid sponging is a nursing practice which may help to reduce this problem.

The patient's body temperature is assessed and recorded prior to and following this nursing practice to evaluate the effect of the tepid sponge.

Mobilising

Patient movements prior to, during and following the tepid sponge should be kept to a minimum as body temperature is lowest during periods of relative inactivity.

Sleeping

An environment conducive to resting and sleeping should be provided throughout the day to further decrease the patient's activity.

Suggested reading   Boore J, Champion R, Ferguson M (eds) 1987 Nursing the physically ill adult. Churchill
Livingstone, Edinburgh, pp 883–888
Brunner L, Suddarth D 1985 The Lippincott manual of medical–surgical nursing,
Volume 1. Harper & Row, London, p 40
Perry A, Rotter P 1986 Clinical nursing skills and techniques. C. V. Mosby, St Louis, pp
152–155
Roper N, Logan W, Tierney A 1990 The elements of nursing, 3rd edn. Churchill
Livingstone, Edinburgh, pp 236–238

Mobilising

Lifting, Turning and Moving Patients

Objectives

By the end of this section you should know how to:

- assess the requirements correctly
- plan the safest method of moving the patient
- adapt the principles of movement to suit each particular situation

Related information

Revision of the anatomy and physiology of the spinal column and main joints and muscles of the body.

Revision of the current theories on safe and efficient lifting and handling practices (particularly the articles by Vasey & Crozler in Suggested reading).

Some indications for lifting a patient

It may be necessary for one, two or more staff, with the help of mechanical aids, to lift a patient when he is unable to move himself because of:

- severe injury
- major surgery
- paralysis
- acute illness
- weakness
- unconsciousness

Figure 8.1
Centre of gravity

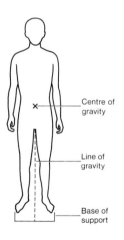

Centre of gravity

Line of gravity

Base of support

Outline of the procedure

It is important to understand the theories of safe and efficient lifting and handling practices. In normal adults the imaginary 'centre of gravity' point is near the base of the spine. If suspended from this point, in theory, the body would balance (Fig 8.1). The feet form what is called the 'base' and if the centre of gravity moves beyond the area of the base, the body will become unbalanced and fall unless all the major muscles of the trunk and legs tense and hold the body upright. A prolonged period of imbalance or 'top heavy' action can lead to stress and strain of these muscles and ultimately injury and pain (Fig 8.2). Widening of the base to keep the centre of gravity within the baseline will help to avoid this.

When preparing to lift, collapse the spine, relax the knees and widen the base appropriately. Approach the load to be lifted with open palms and hold from underneath upwards to avoid pinching grips on the load and unnecessary stress on the muscles of the fingers, hands and arms. Hold the load as near to your body as possible. Just before the 'effort' phase of the lift, recollapse the spine so that the lift begins from a moving position, then lead with the top of the head in the direction of the lift and reform the spine. The momentum caused by this action should allow the patient to come with you. If necessary, break the lift into several stages, repositioning yourself after each move.

Figure 8.2
Examples of safe and unsafe
lifting

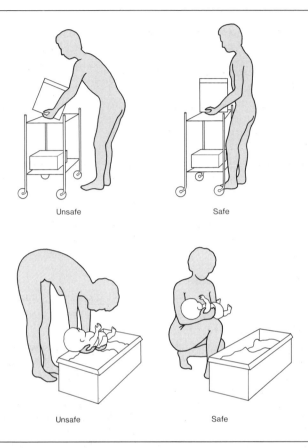

Unsafe   Safe

Unsafe   Safe

Equipment   Mechanical aids, e.g. lifting device (Fig 8.3), turning circle aid

Figure 8.3
Using a mechanical aid to lift a
patient into a bath

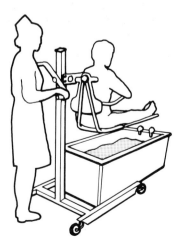

Guidelines for this nursing practice

- assess the requirements with regard to the condition of the patient and his weight, the number of helpers, the most appropriate type of lift, the lifting environment

- clear the area, if possible, of any obstacles

- ensure appropriate bed height

- collect any help or mechanical aids required

- explain fully to the patient and any helpers what is going to happen and what is expected of them

- observe the patient throughout this activity

- adopt a suitable position for the lift or manoeuvre any mechanical aid into position for the lift

- apply the recommended theories of safe and efficient lifting and handling practices when performing the lift, to protect nursing staff from back injury

- carry out the lift, with one nurse acting as the leader and giving instructions

- ensure that the patient is left feeling as comfortable as possible

There should always be a minimum of two nurses to lift patients. They should:

Australian or shoulder lift

This method of lifting is recommended if possible. Research has demonstrated that this lift produces significantly lower intra-abdominal pressure in the lifter than any of the others.

The patient is helped to sit upright in bed and both nurses stand level with the patient's hips. The nurses collapse their spines and widen their base, pointing the foot nearest the top of the bed in the direction of the lift. The shoulder nearest the patient is placed firmly under his axilla so that his arms rest on the nurses' backs. The arms of the shoulder which is pressing into the patient's axilla are placed as high up under the patient's thighs as possible. Approaching each other with open hands, the nurses secure a fastening clasp on each other's arm about wrist level. The nurses' free hand can be placed on the bed above the patient, providing extra support for the 'effort phase' of the lift. The leader gives the start signal and the nurses begin the 'effort phase' of the lift by leading with the top of their heads, reforming their spines and transferring their weight to their forward foot. They carry the patient with them and collapse their spines again to put the patient back down on the bed in the new position. The patient is left feeling as comfortable as possible (Fig. 8.4).

Figure 8.4
Two nurses lifting a patient in bed: Australian lift (Adapted from Roper N, Logan W, Tierney A 1990 The elements of nursing, 3rd edn. Churchill Livingstone, Edinburgh)

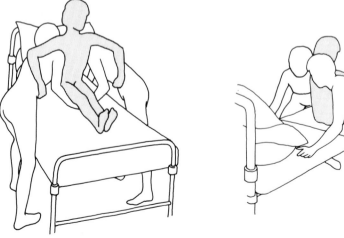

Guidelines for this
nursing practice
continued

Orthodox lift

This lift produces greater intra-abdominal pressure in the lifter, but is sometimes the lift of choice when the patient is unable to cooperate sufficiently to allow the shoulder lift to be performed. The nurses face each other on either side of the patient. They collapse their spines and widen their base, pointing the leading foot in the direction in which it is going to move. The arms nearest the top of the bed are put round the patient's back as low down as possible and approaching the patient's waistline with an open hand, a suitable fastening position is found. The other arms are similarly fixed under the patient's thighs, as near his buttocks as possible. The patient is asked to cross his arms over his chest. The leader gives the signal and the lifters reform their spines, leading with the top of their heads and transferring the weight to their leading feet, carrying the patient with them. They collapse their spines again to put the patient back down on the bed. The patient is left feeling as comfortable as possible (Fig. 8.5).

Figure 8.5
Two nurses lifting a patient in bed: orthodox lift (Adapted from Roper N, Logan W, Tierney A 1990 The elements of nursing, 3rd edn. Churchill Livingstone, Edinburgh)

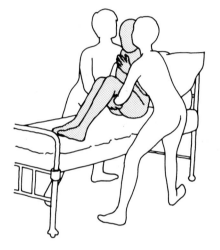 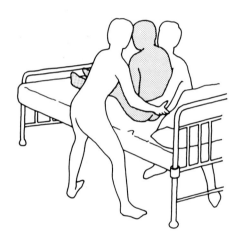

Relevance to the activities of living

Maintaining a safe environment

The safety of the patient and of nursing staff is of equal importance. To avoid the danger of back injury to staff, mechanical aids should be used on all possible occasions.

Know your own lifting capacity and do not exceed it. Do not lift unnecessarily. If something goes wrong with the lift do not be afraid to lower the patient gently to the floor. Make him comfortable and summon help.

Communicating

Good communication between the lifters, and between the lifters and the patient, is very important for successful movement which does no harm to the lifters or the patient.

Successful communication will enable the patient to feel safer and more confident in the nurses' lifting abilities.

Personal cleansing and dressing

Appropriate clothing and footwear for nurses and patient can help the success of a lifting manoeuvre.

Mobilising

Patients should be encouraged to help move themselves as much as possible. Sometimes nurses lift patients unnecessarily because it is quicker than waiting for the patient to move himself.

Suggested reading

Boore J, Champion R, Ferguson M (eds) 1987 Nursing the physically ill adult. Churchill Livingstone, Edinburgh, pp 291–296

Farmer P 1987 Mechanical aids. Nursing Times 82(28) July 15: 36–37

Hawkey B, Clarke M 1990 Dress sense or nonsense. Nursing Times 86(3) January 17: 28–31

Hayne C 1985 Safe patient movement: an alternative approach. Nursing 2(33) January: 960

Lloyd P et al 1987 The handling of patients, 2nd edn. Back Pain Association and R.C.N. London: p 55

Roper N, Logan W, Tierney A 1990 The elements of nursing, 3rd edn. Churchill Livingstone, Edinburgh

Scholey M 1982 The shoulder lift. Nursing Times 78(12) March 24: 506–507

Tarling C 1985 Aids to patient mobility. Nursing 2(33) January: 974

Thompson C 1987 Learning to lift. Nursing Times 83(15) April 15: 34–35

Vasey J, Crozier L 1982 A neuromuscular approach.
1. A move in the right direction. Nursing Mirror 154(17) April 28: 42–47
2. Get into condition. Nursing Mirror 154(18) May 5: 22–28
3. At ease. Nursing Mirror 154(19) May 12: 28–31
4. Handle with care. Nursing Mirror 154(20) May 19: 30–32
5. Easy on the base. Nursing Mirror 154(21) May 26: 36–42
6. Safety first. Nursing Mirror 154(22) June 2: 44–48

Active and Passive Exercises

Objectives

By the end of this section you should know how to:

- prepare the patient for this nursing practice
- carry out active and passive exercises

Related information

Revision of the anatomy and physiology of the musculoskeletal system.

Some indications for active and passive exercises

Active and passive exercises (Fig. 8.6) are muscle and joint movements carried out to assist circulation, maintain muscle tone and prevent the development of joint contracture. These exercises can be performed by the patient (active) or by the nurse helping the patient (passive) and are indicated:

- following an anaesthetic and surgery
- during a period of unconsciousness
- during reduced mobility such as bedrest

Figure 8.6
Passive (assisted) exercises for the bedfast patient (Reproduced with permission from Roper N, Logan W, Tierney A 1985 The elements of nursing, 2nd edn. Churchill Livingstone, Edinburgh)

Spine Cervical

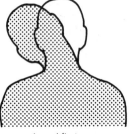

Lateral flexion

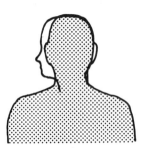

Rotation

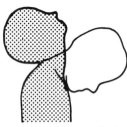

Hyperextension   Flexion

Trunk

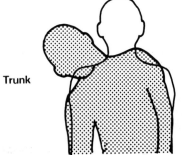

Lateral flexion

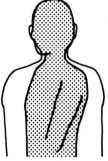

Rotation

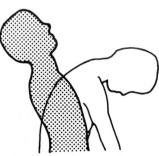

Hyperextension   Flexion

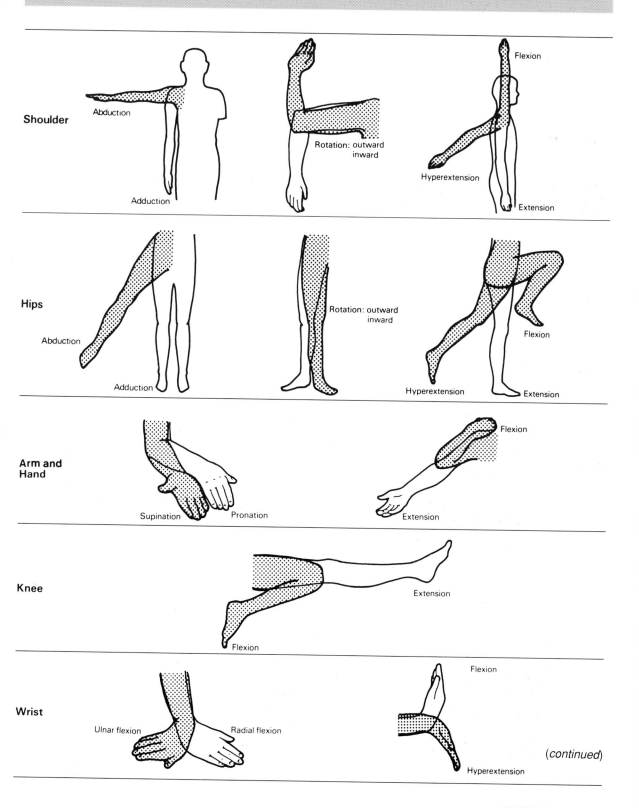

Shoulder

Abduction

Adduction

Rotation: outward
inward

Flexion

Hyperextension

Extension

Hips

Abduction

Adduction

Rotation: outward
inward

Flexion

Hyperextension

Extension

Arm and Hand

Supination   Pronation

Flexion

Extension

Knee

Extension

Flexion

Wrist

Ulnar flexion   Radial flexion

Flexion

Hyperextension

(continued)

Active and Passive Exercises

Figure 8.4 *continued*

Ankle

Eversion   Inversion

Dorsiflexion

Plantar flexion

Fingers

Separated

Together

Extension

Flexion

Toes

Together

Separated

Extension

Flexion

Guidelines for this nursing practice

- explain the nursing practice to the patient and gain his consent and cooperation
- ensure the patient's privacy
- observe the patient throughout this activity
- wash the hands
- help the patient into a comfortable position. The patient's position may require to be altered during the nursing practice

- assist the patient to move the cervical spine and trunk through the normal range of movement for that patient
- taking each limb separately, assist the patient to move all the joints of the limb through the normal range of movement for that patient
- ensure that the patient is left feeling as comfortable as possible
- document the nursing practice appropriately, monitor after-effects and report abnormal findings immediately

Relevance to the activities of living

Maintaining a safe environment

To prevent cross-infection the nurse should wash her hands before commencing and on completion of the nursing practice.

Communicating

The nurse should give an easily understood explanation to the patient as to the importance of performing the active and/or passive exercises. When appropriate the nurse should help to teach the patient to perform the exercises independently.

The patient should not suffer any discomfort when regularly performing active or passive exercises unless there is an underlying disease or a developing complication.

Breathing

Active and passive exercises have the benefit of increasing the patient's depth and rate of respiration, which may help to prevent the development of a chest infection during his period of reduced mobility.

The exercises can assist venous circulation, preventing venous stasis which can cause deep vein thrombosis. Benefit of the exercises may also be enhanced by the use of anti-embolic stockings and/or administration of subcutaneous heparin. Pulmonary embolism is a serious complication, occasionally fatal, following the development of a deep vein thrombosis, therefore the exercise pattern should be performed regularly.

Mobilising

Assisting the patient with active and passive exercises is the dual responsibility of the physiotherapist and the nurse.

Exercise helps to maintain muscle tone and movement so that when the patient's normal range of mobility can be resumed no joint stiffness or muscle weakness will hinder mobilisation. Joints or muscle tissue should never be forced through any movement, as this could cause injury, with a resultant effect on the range of mobility.

When the nurse performs passive exercises, the joints and muscles not being exercised must be well supported otherwise injury will occur.

Exercising a paralysed limb may help to prevent joint and/or muscle contracture which would interfere with the patient's already reduced mobility.

Suggested reading

Drinkwater K 1989 Management of deep vein thrombosis. Surgical Nurse 2(1) February: 24–26
Green S, Wickenden A 1982 Deep vein thrombosis. Nursing 1(33) January: 1468–1469
Love C 1990 Deep vein thrombosis.
1. Threat to recovery. Nursing Times 86(5) January 31: 40–43
2. Methods of prevention. Nursing Times 86(6) February 7: 52–55
Roper N, Logan W, Tierney A 1990 The elements of nursing, 3rd edn. Churchill Livingstone, Edinburgh, pp 259–263

Section 9

Expressing Sexuality

Vaginal Examination

Objectives

By the end of this section you should know how to:

- prepare the patient for this procedure
- collect and prepare the equipment
- describe the various positions which enable this examination to be carried out most easily
- assist the medical practitioner as necessary

Related information

Revision of the anatomy and physiology of the female reproductive system.

Some indications for a vaginal examination

The vagina can be examined visually or digitally for the following reasons:

- to assess the position, size, texture or appearance of the cervix and vagina
- to obtain a swab from the cervix or vagina
- to obtain a cervical smear for cytological examination
- to administer treatment to the cervix or vagina
- to determine the site of a haemorrhage

Outline of the procedure

The medical practitioner puts on a pair of disposable gloves and applies some water-soluble lubricant to the dominant hand. He then inserts two or three fingers of the dominant hand into the vagina and palpates the uterus through the abdominal wall with the non-dominant hand. This is known as a *digital* or *bimanual* examination.

For a *visual* examination of the vagina and cervix the medical practitioner will insert a lubricated speculum – usually a Sims' or Cusco's – into the vagina (Fig. 9.1). He opens the speculum to separate the vaginal walls to enable inspection of the vagina and cervix, and to do this a good light is required. He may use a pair of vulsellum forceps to hold the cervix while he examines it. A pair of swab-holding forceps and some swabs may be necessary to wipe away any blood or vaginal discharge which might be obstructing inspection of the mucosa. To obtain a cervical smear, he scrapes the cervix with the cervical spatula and smears the products onto a microscopic slide, which is then put into a container with fixative and dispatched to cytology for examination. After the examination he closes the speculum and removes it gently from the vagina.

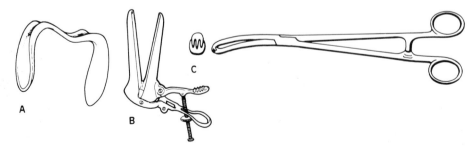

Figure 9.1
Examples of vaginal specula
A Sims'
B Cusco's
C Vulsellum
(Figs. A and B reproduced with permission from Chilman A, Thomas M (eds) 1987 Understanding nursing care, 3rd edn. Churchill Livingstone, Edinburgh)

A

B

C

Equipment

Tray or trolley

For digital examination:
— disposable gloves
— water-soluble lubricant
— receptacle for soiled disposables

For visual examination, in addition to the above:
— sterile vaginal speculum
— sterile vulsellum forceps
— sterile swab-holding forceps
— swabs
— light source
— cervical spatula (Ayre's) or cervical brush (Fig. 9.2)
— glass slide
— container with fixative
— completed laboratory form and plastic specimen bag for safe transport

Figure 9.2
A Cervical spatulae (Ayre's)
B Cervical brush

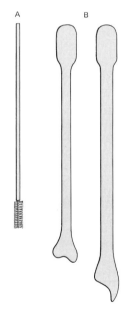

A   B

The position of the patient

There are several suitable positions for this procedure. The position of choice is usually the one most convenient for the medical practitioner and the patient:

The recumbent position: the patient lies on her back with her knees drawn up and separated and the sides of her feet resting on the bed (Fig. 9.3).

The left lateral position: the patient lies on her left side with her knees flexed and her buttocks near the edge of the bed.

The knee–chest position: the patient kneels on the bed with her thighs vertical. Her head is turned to one side and her chest rests on a pillow.

The lithotomy position: the patient's buttocks are at the end of the table or couch. The thighs are flexed on the trunk and the legs flexed on the thighs. Supports attached to the table or couch keep the patient's legs in the correct position. To avoid injury to the patient, both legs must be lifted gently into position at the same time (Fig. 9.3).

Figure 9.3
Two common positions used for vaginal examination
A Recumbent position
B Lithotomy position

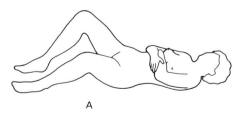
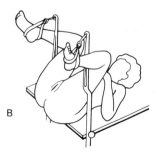

A   B

Guidelines for this nursing practice

- help to explain the procedure to the patient and gain her consent and cooperation
- ensure as much privacy as possible for the patient
- collect and prepare the equipment
- assist the patient into the agreed position
- observe the patient throughout this activity
- assist the medical practitioner and the patient as necessary

- ensure that the patient is left feeling as comfortable as possible afterwards
- dispose of the equipment safely
- dispatch any specimens to the laboratory with the completed form and in a plastic specimen bag
- document this procedure, monitor after-effects and report abnormal findings immediately

Relevance to the activities of living

Maintaining a safe environment

Nowadays, medical practitioners are advised to use a disposable vaginal speculum to prevent any possibility of infecting staff or subsequent patients with HIV which causes the disease condition AIDS. Because of the current limited knowledge about HIV, the nurse should wear disposable gloves when there is a risk of contact with vaginal discharge or soiled equipment.

Communicating

If the patient can cooperate by relaxing as much as possible, it makes it easier for the medical practitioner to carry out this examination. A clear explanation of why the examination is necessary and how the patient can relax, e.g. by deep breathing, will help to ensure relaxation.

Breathing

Slow, regular, concentrated deep breathing will help the patient to relax the abdominal and perineal muscles.

Eliminating

The patient should be given the opportunity to empty her bladder before the examination. This makes it easier for the medical practitioner to palpate the uterus, and it is more comfortable for the patient, who is usually feeling apprehensive.

Personal cleansing and dressing

If treatment is to be given during the examination which may result in vaginal discharge, the patient should have prior information so that appropriate underwear will be worn.

Expressing sexuality

Many patients find this examination stressful and embarrassing. The best privacy possible should be provided and the patient should be covered as much as possible. The examination should be carried out with the surroundings as calm and relaxed as possible.

Suggested reading

Couch-Hockedy S 1989 Women's experience of gynaecology. Professional Nurse 4(4) January: 173–175

Gregory S, McKie L 1990 Smear tactics. Nursing Times 86(19) May 9: 38–40

Hamilton H (ed) 1985 Nurse's reference library – procedures. Springhouse Corporation, Pennsylvania, pp 724–726

Hunter C 1985 Easing the tension. Nursing Times 81(3) January 16: 40–43

Lui D 1988 Management approaches in menorrhagia. British Journal of Sexual Medicine July: 10–13

Nicholson J 1989 Smear campaign. Nursing Times 85(13) March 29: 40–42 (effect of repeat smears on patients)

Roper N, Logan W, Tierney A 1990 The elements of nursing, 3rd edn. Churchill Livingstone, Edinburgh, pp 303–305

Sadler C 1989 The unmet gynaecological needs of older women. Nursing 3(47) December: 34

Sadler C 1989 Breast screening. Nursing 3(45) November: 35

Vaginal Pessaries

Objectives

By the end of this section you should know how to:

- prepare the patient for this nursing practice
- collect and prepare the equipment
- administer the prescribed pessaries to the patient

Related information

Revision of the anatomy and physiology of the cervix and vagina.

Some indications for administering medicinal vaginal pessaries

Vaginal pessaries are cones or cylinders of medication which are inserted into the vagina, where they dissolve and have their effect topically or by absorption. They are used:

- to administer medication, e.g. antibiotics

Equipment

Tray
Prescribed pessaries
Disposable gloves
Water-soluble lubricant
Protective pad
Receptacle for soiled disposables

Guidelines for this nursing practice

- explain the nursing practice to the patient to gain her consent and cooperation
- collect, check and prepare the equipment
- ensure maximum privacy and assist the patient into the position agreed by her and the nurse. See Vaginal examination for a description of suitable positions (p. 305)
- observe the patient throughout this activity
- lubricate the end of the pessary
- put on the disposable gloves
- part the labia majora with the non-dominant hand, and on locating the vagina insert the pessary in an upwards and backwards direction with the dominant hand for the length of the index finger if possible
- put a protective pad over the patient's vulval area to protect the patient's underwear from being stained by the dissolving pessary
- ensure the patient is left feeling as comfortable as possible
- dispose of the equipment safely
- document this nursing practice appropriately, monitor after-effects and report abnormal findings immediately

Relevance to the activities of living

Maintaining a safe environment

Although this does not require aseptic technique, the equipment should be disposable and the nurse should wash her hands before commencing and on completion of the nursing practice.

Communicating

A clear explanation should be given to gain the patient's consent and cooperation, which should make the administering of the pessary easier.

Eliminating

The patient should be given the opportunity to empty her bowel and bladder before the pessary is administered. This gives the pessary time to dissolve and be absorbed before the patient's next visit to the toilet.

Mobilising

It should be suggested to the patient that she moves around as little as possible for half an hour after the insertion of the pessary, so that it can dissolve and be absorbed.

Expressing sexuality

This can be an embarrassing practice for some patients and maximum privacy is important.

Suggested reading

Bailey R, Grayson J 1983 Obstetric and gynaecological nursing. Baillière Tindall, London, pp 233–234, 332–333

Masling J 1988 Menopause: a change for the better? Nursing Times 84(39) September 28: 35–38

Reynolds M 1984 Gynaecological nursing. Blackwell Scientific Publications, Oxford, pp 30–33, 127–128

Roper N, Logan W, Tierney A 1990 The elements of nursing, 3rd edn. Churchill Livingstone, Edinburgh, p 306

Sleeping

The Unconscious Patient

Objectives

By the end of this section you should know how to:

- maintain an adequate airway for the unconscious patient
- care for the unconscious patient in such a way that his activities of living are appropriately maintained despite almost total dependency

Related information

Revision of the anatomy and physiology of the nervous system with special reference to the brain.

Review of health authority policy related to the care of the unconscious patient.

Some indications for care during a state of unconsciousness

Nursing intervention is required when a patient's level of consciousness is such that, unaided, he can no longer maintain a clear airway; his normal protective reflexes are so reduced that he can no longer maintain the safety of his environment; and he is unable to perform everyday activities of living.

The unconscious state is most commonly associated with:

- patients who have a cerebral vascular accident, e.g.:
  — cerebral haemorrhage
  — cerebral embolus or ischaemia
  — subarachnoid haemorrhage
- patients who have taken an overdose of analgesic drugs
- patients who have a traumatic head injury
- patients who have a brain tumour
- patients who are in a comatosed state caused by:
  — severe infection
  — hypothermia
  — uncontrolled diabetes mellitus (hyperglycaemia or hypoglycaemia)
- patients who have received anaesthetic medication during and following surgery

Equipment

Bed with a detachable head
Padded cot sides
Guedel disposable airway
Ambubag with valve and mask
Equipment for assessing level of consciousness
Equipment for oral, pharyngeal or tracheal suction
Equipment for oxygen therapy
Equipment for nasogastric feeding
Mouth care tray
Eye care tray
Catheter care tray
Equipment for endotracheal intubation if required
(Details of the equipment for specific nursing practices can be found in the relevant sections of this book)

Equipment for assessing the level of consciousness

Pencil torch to assess eye pupil size and reaction

Consciousness level chart, e.g. Glasgow coma scale

The Glasgow Coma Scale enables the assessment of level of consciousness to be made, using a numbered scale. The assessment is of motor activity, e.g. limb movements, verbal responses, reaction to pain, and pupil reactions to light (Fig. 10.1, p. 314). This scale is now used in many health authorities and each area may have documentation of the scale of recordings presented in a different way, and may incorporate other recordings on the same chart. This has been allowed without any infringement of copyright.

Guidelines for this nursing practice

The most important aspect of nursing is the maintenance of a clear airway while the reason for the patient's unconsciousness is diagnosed and treated.

- remove any dentures which may be present and could obstruct the airway

- turn the patient into a semi-prone position or on to his side, with his neck extended to prevent the tongue from slipping back and occluding the airway. This will also prevent any secretions from flowing into the trachea when the swallowing reflex is absent

- observe the patient throughout this activity

- perform oral and pharyngeal suction, or endotracheal suction if appropriate (see Tracheal suction, p. 142)

- insert a plastic airway if required, to help maintain an adequate airway

- administer oxygen therapy as prescribed

- position the patient's limbs to maintain his position comfortably and to allow an adequate flow of blood circulation to all his extremities

- assess and record the level of consciousness every 2 hours

- perform oral and pharyngeal suction every 2 hours or as frequently as required, either directly or through the airway as appropriate

- change the position of the patient to alternate sides every 2 hours to maintain healthy tissue at pressure areas and to aid the expansion of each lung (see Pressure area/Skin care, p. 256)

- provide all nursing care as frequently as required, explaining the care to the patient despite his unconscious state and ensuring his privacy before commencing

- record the temperature, pulse, respiration rates and blood pressure as frequently as required

- document all nursing practices appropriately and report abnormal findings immediately

Figure 10.1

Glasgow Coma Scale: chart for documenting assessment of patient's level of consciousness

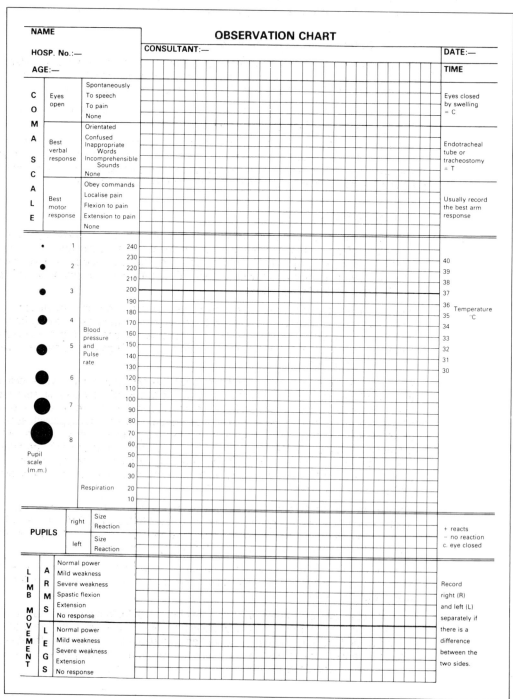

Relevance to the activities of living

A patient who is unconscious is at or near the totally dependent end of the dependence – independence continuum. Nursing staff have to assist, or perform for him, the various activities of living until he fully regains consciousness.

Maintaining a safe environment

The patient should be nursed on a firm bed in an area where he can be constantly observed. This may mean a single cubicle with a nurse to provide special care, or a bed near the nurses' station where frequent observations can be maintained.

The area should be well lit so that any change in the patient's colour can be noted, and abnormal findings reported.

Cot sides should be in position except when nursing practices are being performed. This will prevent the patient from falling if he is restless or in a semiconscious state. The cot sides should be padded to prevent the patient damaging himself on any hard equipment, and pillows placed appropriately can be used effectively.

Communicating

The level of consciousness should be assessed 2-hourly or as ordered by the medical practitioner. Before beginning the assessment the nurse should ensure that the patient is as comfortable as possible in the cicumstances. The response to verbal commands, and the movement of limbs may be impaired if the patient is uncomfortable or in pain, which may also affect pupil reactions.

It is essential to make sure that the patient has no major problem of deafness. A profoundly deaf patient will not respond to any verbal instructions, and may be less comatosed than the nurse realises. He may become restless and frightened when regaining consciousness as explanations of his surroundings and nursing interventions have not been heard.

A nursing assessment of the patient should be obtained from his family, especially if the patient is unconscious on admission, and this should also include his social and family background. It is a great help to communication if the nurse knows the patient's forename or nickname as he may not readily respond to a formal approach such as 'Mr Smith'. It is also a help to know something about the patient's family and interests. Individualised care is enhanced when the nurse is able to chat about the grandchildren, or the dog, or the latest pop records even when there is no immediate response from the patient. This also helps the family to feel that the nursing remains individualised and personal.

The nurse should talk to the patient at every opportunity, even if he appears deeply unconscious. She should try to orientate the patient to his surroundings even where there appears to be no response. He should be told where he is and why; and should be told what day it is, and the date and time as appropriate.

Before commencing any nursing intervention the nurse should introduce herself and explain what is to happen, and should continue to reinforce this throughout the time she is with the patient.

The use of touch as a means of communication is helpful to both the patient and the nurse when caring for the unconscious patient. Physical contact with friends or relatives can help to reorientate a patient as he regains consciousness. Relatives should be encouraged to sit beside an unconscious patient and hold his hand as well as talk to him, whenever they visit.

Relevance to the
activities of living
continued

The patient's response to pain should be noted as part of the assessment of the level of consciousness. This can be done by squeezing the lobes of the ears, squeezing the back of the heel on each side of the achilles tendon, or applying pressure to the fingernail bed. None of these actions will cause damage to the patient but he will react if he feels the pressure as pain. The way his limbs move in response to pain should be noted and recorded on the assessment chart.

Eye care should be carried out 2-hourly. The inability to blink prevents the eyes from being bathed in lacrimal fluid, and the unconscious patient is at risk of developing corneal ulcers if the eyes are not treated regularly (see Eye care, p. 52).

The nursing plan should indicate how and when nursing care is carried out, and should include the position of the patient for each period of turning.

Breathing

A clear airway should be maintained until the patient has fully recovered consciousness and has an adequate swallowing and cough reflex.

The respiration rate should be recorded as frequently as necessary, but at least every 4 hours. The depth and the pattern of respiration should also be noted, as well as any evidence of a cough or cough reflex.

The blood pressure and pulse rate should be recorded at least every 4 hours or as frequently as necessary, as any abnormalities may indicate a change in intracranial pressure.

Oral and pharyngeal suction should be performed every 2 hours or as required to clear the airway of secretions. Suction should be performed before turning the patient, as this will prevent secretions from draining into the trachea when he is moved. The amount and consistency of the secretions should be noted and any purulent or blood-stained secretions reported. If the airway is not adequately maintained with routine measures, and the patient has excess secretions which are difficult to clear, the medical practitioner may intubate the trachea with an endotracheal tube, and the patient will breathe through this tube.

The patient's position should be changed 2-hourly, so that he lies on alternate sides. This helps to ensure equal expansion of each lung over 24 hours, and helps with the drainage of any bronchial secretions.

Eating and drinking

Nutrients and fluids have to be given by nasogastric tube or intravenously. The nasogastric route is used when possible, and a nasogastric tube should be passed initially to prevent any inhalation of the stomach contents. When the presence of bowel sounds is established the medical practitioner may prescribe nasogastric feeds (see Enteral feeding, p. 166).

The patient should have frequent mouth care to maintain a healthy oropharyngeal mucosa, and this should be performed every 2 hours (see Mouth care, p. 268).

Fluid intake should be recorded and fluid balance charts maintained to monitor the level of hydration and prevent dehydration.

Eliminating

The unconscious patient is incontinent of both faeces and urine.

Male patients may be fitted with an external sheath catheter, and observations should be maintained for any sign of bladder distension. Catheterisation should be performed for female patients to prevent incontinence increasing the risk of tissue damage to pressure areas. Catheterisation may also be prescribed for male patients who have a prolonged period of unconsciousness.

Catheter care should be performed regularly, and bladder washouts may be prescribed (see Catheterisation, p. 208).

Urinary output should be recorded and fluid balance charts maintained, as this helps to monitor the patient's renal function.

Bowel movements should be noted and recorded. Constipation may be more of a problem than diarrhoea for the unconscious patient, and suppositories or enemas may be prescribed regularly (see Bowel care, p. 218).

Personal cleansing and dressing

The nursing plan should include a daily bed bath and any additional washing as required to keep the patient clean and comfortable and his skin in good condition. The nails should be cut short to prevent abrasions caused by scratching, and his hair should be kept clean and tidy (see Bed bathing, p. 250).

Clothing may have to be adapted to suit the patient's requirements, depending on the reason for his condition. It may not be suitable for him to wear his own clothes, but they should be worn if possible to retain his individuality, and this is often a source of comfort to relatives.

The patient's position should be changed every 2 hours to maintain his skin in good condition (see Skin care p. 256).

Controlling body temperature

The temperature should be recorded 4-hourly, or more frequently as required. Any abnormalities should be reported immediately. Damage to the hypothalamus and its temperature-regulating centre can cause abnormal temperatures to occur.

The bed covers should be adapted to keep the patient comfortably warm. Unconscious patients may show signs of hypothermia, and the nurse should feel the temperature of the feet and hands and note the colour of the skin when observing or working with the patient (see Controlling body temperature, p. 278).

The Unconscious Patient

Relevance to the
activities of living
continued

Mobilising

The unconscious patient should be turned every 2 hours so that the tissues under the pressure areas are kept healthy and the blood circulation is maintained to all areas of the body (see Skin care, p. 256).

Passive exercises should be performed three times a day, under the guidance of the physiotherapist if possible (see Passive exercises, p. 298). This helps to prevent any muscle contractions occurring. In addition, light splints may be applied to the lower limbs for patients who are unconscious for a period of time. These are made individually for each patient by the physiotherapist. If possible the nurse should consult the physiotherapist for guidance on the most suitable method of helping to maintain the patient's musculoskeletal system in good condition, so that when he regains consciousness his mobility is not impaired by any muscular or skeletal abnormalities.

The feet should be supported to prevent drop-foot occurring. This can be done by using well-placed sandbags, but specialised splints or sheepskin bootees are more efficient; the guidance of the physiotherapist is helpful.

The semi-prone position (Fig. 10.2) is the most suitable position for maintaining a clear airway, but it is not so suitable for carrying out various nursing activities. The lateral position is preferable and it is still possible to maintain an adequate airway.

In the lateral position the patient is turned on to his side; his head may be placed on a low pillow with the neck extended. The spine should be extended, and pillows placed at the back to maintain his position. The uppermost leg should be flexed and brought forward to be supported on a pillow clear of the extended lower leg; this prevents internal rotation of the hip and any constriction of blood flow to the lower leg. Pillows should not be placed between the legs. The lower arm should be flexed with the palm facing up and the uppermost arm brought forward and supported on a pillow (Fig. 10.3).

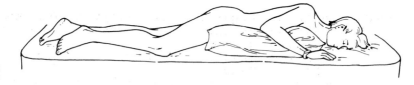

Figure 10.2
Unconscious patient: the semi-prone position (Reproduced with permission from Roper N, Logan W, Tierney A 1985 The elements of nursing, 2nd edn. Churchill Livingstone, Edinburgh)

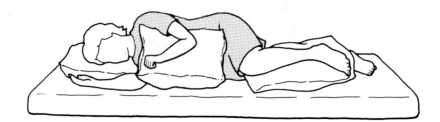

Figure 10.3
Unconscious patient: the lateral position

Working and playing

It is important for the people looking after an unconscious patient to learn as much as possible about his interests; it may even be possible to arrange tapes of his favourite music to be played in an attempt to evoke a response.

When suitable, visits from friends and relatives should be encouraged so that they can talk to him about his hobbies or particular interests.

Expressing sexuality

Although superficially the AL of expressing sexuality may not seem relevant to an unconscious patient, ensuring that, for example, the hair is combed and that a male patient is shaved shows respect for the patient's personal identity and can be of inestimable comfort to the family; in fact, they may wish to assist with these activities.

Sleeping

The nursing of a dependent patient can appear to be constant. If possible any nursing interventions should be arranged to coincide with the time when the patient's position is changed. This is particularly important for patients who show signs of cerebral irritability when handled. It may be beneficial to all unconscious patients to adapt the care so that a period of activity is followed by a long resting period.

Dying

Although an unconscious patient is not necessarily expected to die, the family often associates the apparent unresponsiveness with imminence of death. It is important to listen to the family's concerns, and to explain the cause of unconsciousness and the prognosis, in terms appropriate to the circumstance.

Suggested reading

Allan D 1984 Glasgow Coma scale. Nursing Mirror 158(23) June 13: 32–34

Allan D (ed) 1988 Nursing and the neurosciences. Churchill Livingstone, Edinburgh, ch 4 pp 64–75

De Young S, Grass R B 1987 Coma recovery programme. Rehabilitation Nursing 12(3) May/June: 121–124

Erikson S, Hopkins M A 1987 Grey areas. Informed consent in paediatric and comatose adult patients. Heart Lung 16(3) May: 323–325

Frawley P 1990 Neurological observations. Nursing Times 86(35) August 29: 29–34

Jennett B 1987 Medical aspects of head injury. Medicine International 2(38) February: 1595–1601

Roper N, Logan W, Tierney A 1990 The elements of nursing, 3rd edn. Churchill Livingstone, Edinburgh, pp 328–332

Tosch P 1988 Patients' recollections of their post-traumatic coma. Journal of Neuroscience Nursing 20(5) October: 290–295

Dying

Last Offices

Objectives

By the end of this section you should know how to:

- carry out last offices

Related information

Review of the health authority policy pertaining to last offices.

Revision of bed bathing (see p. 250) and mouth care (see p. 268)

Indication for last offices

Last offices is the nursing care a deceased patient requires before the body is moved to the mortuary.

Equipment

Equipment as for bed bathing (see p. 250)
Equipment as for mouth care (see p. 268)
Incontinence pad or disposable napkin
Dressings pack
Waterproof dressing for open wounds if necessary
Hypoallergenic tape
Shroud
Disposable bowl
2 patient identification bands
Patient identification cards
and/or notification of death cards
} appropriately completed with the patient's full name and other details as requested
Mortuary sheet or clean white sheet
Gauze bandage
Patient clothing list book
Trolley for equipment
Receptacle for patient's clothing
Patient valuables list book
Receptacle for patient's valuables
Receptacle for soiled linen
Receptacle for soiled disposables

Guidelines for this nursing practice

- inform the medical practitioner when a patient is thought to have died
- ensure the patient's privacy and the privacy of relatives, if present
- ensure that either medical or nursing staff notify the patient's relatives of the death, if they are not present
- assist and support bereaved relatives
- inform the nursing officer or deputy, and portering staff
- collect and prepare the equipment
- wash the hands
- remove all upper bed linen leaving a sheet to cover the patient
- lay the patient flat, face up with his limbs in a natural position and his arms by his side
- remove any mechanical aids, e.g. heel pads or rubber rings
- gently close the eyelids
- clean the patient's mouth and replace any dentures
- support the mandible in a closed position using a light pillow. An hour may elapse prior to the continuation of last offices but this is not necessary
- using the disposable bowl manually express the urinary bladder
- remove all tubes and drains unless otherwise instructed
- redress all wounds with a waterproof dressing. When drains or tubes are left in position these should also be covered with a padded waterproof dressing

- wash the patient as for Bed bathing (see p. 250)
- a male patient should be shaved
- all jewellery, once removed, should be listed in the patient valuables book in the presence of two nurses
- apply identification bands and cards to the appropriate limbs and parts of the body
- apply an incontinence pad or disposable napkin
- place the shroud in position
- wrap the body in the sheet, ensuring complete coverage
- secure the sheet with adhesive tape or the gauze bandage
- fix identification card or notification of death card to the sheet using adhesive tape
- list the patient's clothing. Place this clothing and the patient's valuables in a secure place
- dispose of equipment safely
- inform portering staff that the body is ready for collection
- ensure the privacy of the other patients, on arrival of portering staff with the mortuary trolley
- document the nursing practice appropriately

Last Offices

Relevance to the activities of living

Although the patient is deceased, a consideration of the activities of living is important in relation to the family and for the protection of staff.

Maintaining a safe environment

All equipment should be clean or disposable and all precautions be taken to prevent cross-infection. The nurse should wash her hands before commencing and on completion of last offices. On the death of a patient with a contagious disease condition, such as hepatitis B or Acquired Immune Deficiency Syndrome, all isolation techniques should be maintained during last offices. The body is placed in a large polythene bag and sealed, usually with sellotape, prior to being wrapped in a sheet. These practices reduce the risk of infecting nursing, portering and mortuary staff.

If a patient dies unexpectedly or within 24 hours of surgery or within 24 hours of involvement in some form of trauma, the nurse may be requested to leave in position all drains, tubes and dressings during last offices. This may help to establish the cause of death. A patient who dies suddenly and unexpectedly will require a postmortem examination.

Communicating

To communicate with bereaved relatives can be a stressful nursing practice. The nurse should not hide her own feelings of loss and sadness from the deceased's relatives, as the feeling of sharing may be of great support to them. Informing relations adequately and kindly about immediate practicalities is also crucial. For example, it is important that the next of kin understand what is written on the death certificate, and know that it has to be registered locally as only then can funeral arrangements be made.

Following the death of a patient the other patients may question the nurse about the deceased. The nurse should inform the patients kindly and honestly that the patient has died and give support when needed.

The nurse may also require to assist and support her colleagues prior to, during, and following the nursing practice of the last offices.

Dying

The details of practice related to last offices can vary depending on the patient's cultural background and religious practices. The nurse must be aware of the specific requirements prior to, during or following last offices: for example, for the body of the Orthodox Jew there is a ritual purification, no postmortem is permitted, and no organs may be removed for transplant.

The bereaved relatives will require sensitive and compassionate care. Little can be done to ease their distress but the nurse should be aware of the many reactions that may be demonstrated and remain calm and supportive. Any request to see the deceased should be arranged as soon as possible, as this may assist the relatives during the grieving process, and care should be taken to ensure that the patient looks as peaceful as possible, that the environs are cleared of equipment, and that a chair is available.

The deceased person's clothing and valuables should be returned to the next of kin in a sympathetic manner. If clothing and valuables are not able to be returned to the next of kin, they should be transferred to the appropriate administrative department.

Suggested reading

Bell I 1984 Bereavement in continuing care wards. Nursing Times 80(37) September 12: 51–52

Cathcart F 1989 Death: coping with distress. Nursing Times 85(42) October 25: 33–35

Dyne G, Dyne V 1982 Bereavement counselling. Nursing 1(34) February: 1499–1500

Green J 1989 Death with dignity.
1. Islam. Nursing Times 85(5) February 1: 56–57
2. Hinduism. Nursing Times 85(6) February 8: 50–51
3. Sikhism. Nursing Times 85(8) February 15: 56–57
4. Judaism. Nursing Times 85(8) February 22: 64–65
5. Buddhism. Nursing Times 85(9) March 1: 40–41
6. Baha'i Faith. Nursing Times 85(10) March 8: 50–51
7. Funerals abroad. Nursing Times 85(11) March 15: 63

Malcolm D 1985 Letting Alan go (care study of the bereavement process). Nursing Times 81(29) July 17: 30–31

Manley K 1988 The needs and support of relatives. Nursing 3(32) December: 19–22

Neuberger J 1987 Caring for dying people of different faiths. Austen Cornish, London

Roper N, Logan W, Tierney A 1990 The elements of nursing, 3rd edn. Churchill Livingstone, Edinburgh, ch 17

Royal College of Nursing 1981 Verification of death and performance of last offices. Royal College of Nursing, London

Walsh M 1990 Sudden death. Surgical Nurse 3(4) August: 10–13

Walsh M, Ford P 1989 Nursing rituals – research and rational actions. Heinemann Nursing, Oxford, ch 10